Medicinal Mushrooms
A Clinical Guide

Martin Powell

Mycology Press

Copyright © Martin Powell 2010
The right of Martin Powell to be identified as author of this work has been asserted
in accordance with the Copyright, Designs and Patents Act 1988

All rights reserved. No part of this book may be reproduced, stored in a retrieval system,
or transmitted in any form or by any means, electronic, mechanical, photocopying, recording
or otherwise, without the prior permission in writing of the publishers.

First published in 2010 by Mycology Press
The Spinney, Old Willingdon Road, Friston, Eastbourne, East Sussex BN20 0AS U.K.

ISBN 978-0-9566898-0-1

Book Design by CreativeCo Ltd
Big E, 50 Hithercroft Road, Wallingford OX10 9DG

Printed by Butler Tanner & Dennis Ltd
Caxton Road, Frome, Somerset, BA11

Printed on paper made from wood grown in sustainable forests

Contents

Preface 6
Acknowledgements 7
A Note on Mushroom Names 7
Author's Disclaimer 7
Quick Reference Mushrooms 8
Quick Reference Conditions 11

Introduction 14

Members of the Fungal Kingdom 16
Rich Sources of Pharmacologically Active Compounds 17
    Polysaccharides (beta-glucans, proteoglycans and related compounds) 17
    Proteins 19
    Triterpenes 19
    Phenols 20
    Sterols 20
    Chitin 20
    Enzymes 21
Mushroom Polysaccharides - Essential Nutrients for our Immune System? 21
Pharmacokinetics of Mushroom Polysaccharides 24
Th1-Th2, Mushroom Polysaccharides and Immune Balance 25

Understanding Mushroom Products 26

Fruiting Body/Conk/Sclerotium 26
Extracts 26
Spores 27
Mycelium 27
Mycelial Biomass 28
Combination Products 28

Prescribing Medicinal Mushrooms 29

Are there any side effects? 29
Can I use mushroom supplements for patients with
    candidiasis or other fungal conditions? 29
But aren't mushrooms considered Damp in
    traditional Chinese medicine (TCM)? 29
Can mushrooms be taken alongside conventional treatment? 30
Can pregnant or breastfeeding women take medicinal mushrooms? 30

Medicinal Mushrooms   32

Agaricus brasiliensis/Agaricus blazei   32
Antrodia camphorata/Antrodia cinnamomea   36
Armillaria mellea (Honey Mushroom)   39
Auricularia auricula/Auricularia polytricha (Wood Ear)   41
Cordyceps sinensis   43
Flammulina velutipes (Enokitake)   48
Ganoderma lucidum (Reishi)   51
Grifola frondosa (Maitake)   56
Hericium erinaceus (Lion's Mane)   58
Inonotus obliquus (Chaga)   62
Lentinus edodes (Shiitake)   64
Phellinus linteus   67
Pleurotus ostreatus (Oyster Mushroom)   70
Polyporus umbellatus/Grifola umbellata   72
Poria cocos   74
Trametes versicolor/Coriolus versicolor   76
Tremella fuciformis   79

Medicinal Mushrooms in Cancer Therapy   82

Medicinal Mushrooms and Chemotherapy   82
Medicinal Mushrooms and Radiotherapy   84
Medicinal Mushrooms and Surgery   84
Research on Medicinal Mushrooms in Cancer   85
    Bladder Cancer   85
    Brain Cancer   85
    Breast Cancer   85
    Cervical Cancer   87
    Colorectal Cancer   87
    Endometrial Cancer   88
    Gastric Cancer   88
    Leukaemia   88
    Liver Cancer   88
    Lung Cancer   89
    Lymphoma   89
    Ovarian Cancer   89
    Pancreatic Cancer   89
    Prostate Cancer   90
    Skin Cancer   90
Clinical Notes   91

Medicinal Mushrooms for Other Conditions — 96

- Allergic Rhinitis (Hayfever) — 96
- Alzheimers Disease — 96
- Arrythmia — 96
- Asthma — 97
- Bacterial Infections — 97
- Benign Prostatic Hyperplasia (BPH) — 98
- Candidiasis — 98
- Chronic Fatigue Syndrome (CFS - ME) — 99
- Dementia — 100
- Diabetes — 100
- Erectile Dysfunction — 101
- Fluid Retention — 101
- Gastritis — 102
- Hepatitis — 102
- Herpes — 102
- HIV — 103
- HPV — 103
- Hypercholesterolaemia — 104
- Hypertension — 105
- Infertility — 105
- Inflammatory Bowel Disease — 106
- Influenza — 106
- Insomnia/Anxiety — 107
- Kidney Damage — 107
- Liver Damage — 108
- Meniere's Syndrome — 108
- Multiple Sclerosis — 108
- Nerve Damage — 109
- Parkinsons Disease — 109
- Rheumatoid Arthritis — 110
- Systemic Lupus Erythematosus — 110

Appendix, Glossary, Index and Resources — 115

- Medicinal Mushrooms According to Traditional Chinese Medicine — 116
- Glossary — 120
- Index — 125
- Further Reading — 128

Preface

The use of medicinal mushrooms is one of the most exciting areas of natural health, offering significant therapeutic benefit, supported by a long history of traditional use and increasing scientific evidence. However, many questions remain to be addressed if it is to fulfil its potential[1].

In particular the lack of standardisation of mushroom products and lack of comparative clinical research remain significant obstacles to more widespread use.

Given the fact that research has to be paid for, it is perhaps inevitable that most is designed to show the widest range of activity, and therefore sales opportunities, for individual mushroom products, rather than provide the information that clinicians need to decide:

- Which is the best mushroom or combination of mushrooms for my patient?
- What is the best form to give it in - extract or whole mushroom - mycelia or fruiting body?
- What dosage is therapeutically effective?

This book sets out to address these questions and it is my hope that it will assist practitioners and patients alike by providing at least partial answers.

The variable quality of much of the available information, together with the lack of standardisation among mushroom products and the extensive overlap of functionality between different mushrooms, means that there will inevitably be room for differences of opinion regarding the answers to the above questions.

As well as suggesting answers, I have therefore given an overview of the research so that readers can evaluate it for themselves and draw their own conclusions.

In putting the book together I have tried at all times to maximise its usability. A Quick Reference section is included at the beginning with brief summaries of individual mushrooms' main therapeutic application(s) and active constituents, and of the mushroom(s) commonly used for specific conditions, with suggested dosage formats.

In addition to the quick reference section, the book is divided into four parts:

- Introduction to medicinal mushrooms and mushroom products
- Individual monographs on the therapeutic potential of the major medicinal mushrooms
- Discussion of the use of medicinal mushrooms in cancer treatment
- Survey of the clinical application of medicinal mushrooms for other clinical conditions

There is also an appendix on the energetics of mushrooms in traditional Chinese medicine (TCM) for those practitioners trained in this approach.

Acknowledgements

Despite my training as a TCM practitioner, my early attitude to mushrooms was very much shaped by my parents' warning on walks in the forest: 'Don't touch the mushrooms' and I would like to thank Michael Hsieh of Double Crane Enterprises, Taiwan for first introducing me to the therapeutic possibilities of mushrooms and starting me down the road to embracing them.

Many people have helped in the preparation of this book but I would especially like to thank my wife and family for their patient support and tolerance during its preparation, Gao Yufeng for her help with Chinese translation, Professor Godfrey Chan of The University of Hong Kong for his generous permission to use the images on pages 14 and 15, Well Shine Biotechnology (*Antrodia camphorata*), Umberto Pascali (*Armillaria mellea*), Gerhard Schuster (*Polyporus umbellatus*) and Dr Frankie Chan (*Phellinus linteus*) for permission to use their mushroom images and Peter Deadman of the Journal of Chinese Medicine and Jo Dunbar for their suggestions on making the text more accessible.

Lastly I would like to thank the many practitioners who encouraged me in my efforts and to whom this book is dedicated.

A Note on Mushroom Names

Mushroom nomenclature is a complex area with alternative names in use for some medicinal mushrooms and others open to possible future review[1]. Although some mushrooms are more commonly referred to by alternative names (ie. Reishi for *Ganoderma lucidum*), I have decided for the sake of consistency to use the Latin name of each species.

Where alternative Latin names are in use for a given mushroom I have opted for the name used in the International Journal of Medicinal Mushrooms and have noted alternative names where appropriate.

Author's Disclaimer

This book is intended for use by suitably qualified healthcare practitioners. The information it contains is presented for educational use only and is not meant to be a prescription for any disease. If you are experiencing symptoms you are strongly advised to contact a medical doctor or other appropriately qualified healthcare professional.

Martin Powell, Eastbourne
October 2010

Quick Reference – Mushrooms

A note on terminology:

Polysaccharide extract - The term polysaccharide extract is used for convenience although in almost all cases mushroom polysaccharides have bound protein moeities and are also referred to as proteoglycans, or protein-bound polysaccharides. As the typical mushroom polysaccharide is a $(1{\rightarrow}3),(1{\rightarrow}6)$ β-glucan they are also sometimes referred to generically as beta-glucans.

Biomass - This refers to mycelial/young fruiting body biomass, in other words mushroom mycelium cultivated on a grain-based substrate and the resultant 'biomass' (mushroom mycelium and residual substrate) harvested at the point that the mushroom is starting to produce fruiting bodies (the 'primordia' stage). This technique is also referred to as solid-state fermentation.

Mycelium - Refers to mushroom mycelium grown by liquid fermentation (no residual substrate).

For further discussion of different dosage forms, see p.26-28.

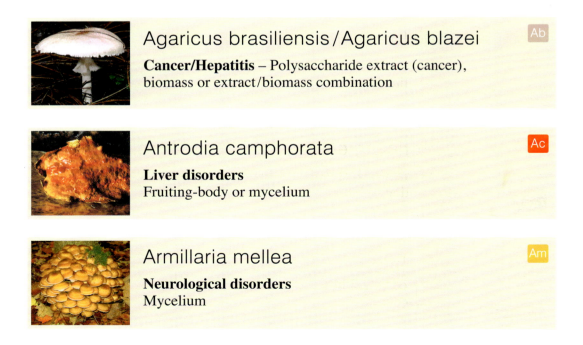

Agaricus brasiliensis/Agaricus blazei — Ab
Cancer/Hepatitis – Polysaccharide extract (cancer), biomass or extract/biomass combination

Antrodia camphorata — Ac
Liver disorders
Fruiting-body or mycelium

Armillaria mellea — Am
Neurological disorders
Mycelium

Auricularia auricula / Auricularia polytricha `Aa`
Cardiovascular support
Polysaccharide extract

Cordyceps sinensis `Cs`
Lung/Liver/Kidney support, infertility/sexual function, diabetes, energy – Biomass

Flammulina velutipes (Enokitake) `Fv`
Cancer prevention, allergies, viral infections
Fruiting body

Ganoderma lucidum (Reishi) `Gl`
Cancer, allergies, insomnia
Triterpene-rich extract

Grifola frondosa (Maitake) `Gf`
Cancer – Polysaccharide extract or polysaccharide extract /fruiting body combination

Hericium erinaceus (Lion's Mane) `He`   M.S.
Dementia, Alzheimers Disease, MRSA
Fruiting body or biomass

Inonotus obliquus (Chaga) `Io`
Cancer, viral infections
Aqueous extract

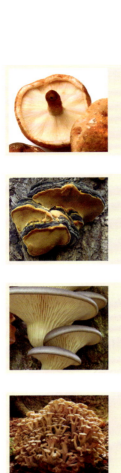

Lentinus edodes (Shiitake) `Le`

Cancer, cholesterol control – Polysaccharide extract (cancer) or fruiting body (cholesterol control)

Phellinus linteus `Pl`

Cancer, autoimmune disorders
Polysaccharide extract

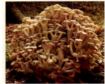

Pleurotus ostreatus (Oyster mushroom) `Po`

Cholesterol control
Fruiting body or biomass

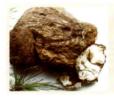

Polyporus umbellatus / Grifola umbellata `Pu`

Cancer, hepatitis, fluid retention – Polysaccharide extract (cancer/hepatitis) or sclerotium (fluid retention)

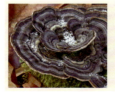

Poria cocos `Pc`

Fluid retention
Sclerotium

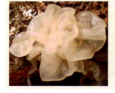

Trametes versicolor / Coriolus versicolor `Tv`

Cancer, CFS/ME, HIV – Polysaccharide extract (cancer), biomass or extract/biomass combination

Tremella fuciformis `Tf`

Cardiovascular/neurological support, radiation exposure
Polysaccharide extract

Quick Reference – Conditions

This is not an exhaustive list of every mushroom that can be used for every condition, or of every dosage form that may be beneficial, but rather of which mushrooms and which dosage forms are most relevant for each condition. A fuller discussion of each condition is included in the last section, or in some cases under the mushroom entry itself.

[Ps] - For several conditions the beneficial effect of medicinal mushrooms is largely due to the ability of **mushroom polysaccharides** (beta-glucans/proteoglycans etc.) to modulate and increase the cytotoxic efficacy of our immune response. In these cases the fact that one mushroom or one dosage form shows efficacy does not mean that other mushrooms would not be at least as effective, or that dosage forms with higher concentrations of polysaccharides would not be more effective.

Without clear evidence for superior activity of a single mushroom it can be beneficial, given the increased immunological activity of multi-mushroom formulae, to use combinations of polysaccharide extracts from several mushrooms (*see combination products, p.28*).

Allergic Rhinitis (Hayfever) [Gl]

- *Ganoderma lucidum* - extract (triterpene-rich) - 1-3g/day

Alzheimers Disease [He] [Gl]

- *Hericium erinaceus* - fruiting body or biomass - 3-5g/day
- *Ganoderma lucidum* - extract - 1-3g/day

Anti-aging [Gl] [Cs] [Tf]

- *Ganoderma lucidum* - extract (triterpene-rich) - 1-3g/day
- *Cordyceps sinensis* - biomass - 1-3g/day
- *Tremella fuciformis* - polysaccharide extract - 1-3g/day

Arrythmia [Cs]

- *Cordyceps sinensis* - biomass - 3-6g/day

Asthma [Cs] [Gl]

- *Cordyceps sinensis* - biomass - 3g/day
- *Ganoderma lucidum* - extract (triterpene-rich) - 1-3g/day

Benign Prostatic Hyperplasia (BPH)

- *Ganoderma lucidum* - extract (triterpene-rich) - 1-3g/day

Cancer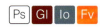

All medicinal mushrooms show anti-cancer properties with large scale clinical trials of *Trametes versicolor* and *Lentinus edodes*, and on a smaller scale, *Grifola frondosa*, *Ganoderma lucidum* and *Agaricus brasiliensis*. All clinical trials have used polysaccharide extracts. There is some evidence that combinations of mushrooms may have higher activity.

- Polysaccharide extracts - 3-6g/day
- *Ganoderma lucidum* - extract (triterpene-rich) - 3-6g/day
- *Inonotus obliquus* - aqueous extract - 2-5g/day
- *Flammulina velutipes* (prevention) - fruiting body - 3-5g/day

Candidiasis

- *Lentinus edodes* - biomass - 2-3g/day
- *Trametes versicolor* - biomass - 2-3g/day

Cardiovascular Support

- *Tremella fuciformis* - polysaccharide extract - 1-3g/day

Chronic Fatigue Syndrome (CFS - ME)

- Polysaccharide extracts - 1-3g/day
- *Trametes versicolor* - biomass - 3g/day

Dementia

- *Hericium erinaceus* - fruiting body or biomass - 3-5g/day

Diabetes

- *Cordyceps sinensis* - biomass - 3-5g/day

Erectile Dysfunction

- *Cordyceps sinensis* - biomass - 3g/day

Fluid Retention

- *Polyporus umbellatus* - sclerotium - 6-15g/day

Gastritis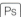

- *Hericium erinaceus* fruiting body or biomass - 25g/day

Hepatitis

- Polysaccharide extracts - 1.5-3g/day
- *Cordyceps sinensis* - biomass - 3g/day

Herpes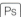

- Polysaccharide extracts - 1-3g/day

HIV

- Polysaccharide extracts - 1-3g/day
- *Trametes versicolor* - biomass - 3-6g/day
- *Inonotus obliquus* - aqueous extract - 2-5g/day

HPV

- Polysaccharide extracts - 1-3g/day
- *Trametes versicolor* - biomass - 3g/day

Hypercholesterolaemia

- *Pleurotus ostreatus* - fruiting body - 15-20g/day
- *Lentinus edodes* - fruiting body or biomass - 9-15g/day

Hypertension

- *Ganoderma lucidum* - triterpene-rich extract - 2-6g/day

Infertility

- *Cordyceps sinensis* - biomass - 3g/day

Inflammatory Bowel Disease

- Polysaccharide extracts - 2-6g/day

Influenza

- Polysaccharide extracts - 1-3g/day

Insomnia/Anxiety

- *Ganoderma lucidum* - triterpene-rich extracts - 1-3g/day

Kidney Damage

- *Cordyceps sinensis* - biomass - 3g/day

Liver Damage

- *Cordyceps sinensis* - biomass - 3g/day
- *Ganoderma lucidum* - triterpene-rich extracts - 1-3g/day
- *Antrodia camphorata* - fruiting body 1g/day or mycelium 1-3g/day

Meniere's Syndrome

- *Armillaria mellea* - mycelium - 3-5g/day

MRSA

- *Hericium erinaceus* - fruiting body or biomass - 25-50g/day

Multiple Sclerosis

- *Hericium erinaceus* - fruiting body or biomass - 3-5g/day

Nerve Damage

- *Hericium erinaceus* - fruiting body or biomass - 3-5g/day
- *Ganoderma lucidum* - sporoderm-broken spores - 1-3g/day

Parkinson's Disease

- *Ganoderma lucidum* - triterpene-rich extracts - 1-3g/day
- *Flammulina velutipes* - fruiting body - 3-5g/day

Rheumatoid Arthritis

- *Phellinus linteus* - polysaccharide extract - 3g/day
- *Ganoderma lucidum* - triterpene-rich extract - 3g/day

Smoking

- *Tremella fuciformis* - polysaccharide extract - 3g/day

Systemic Lupus Erythematosus

- *Antrodia camphorata* - mycelium - 3-6g/day

Introduction

Mushrooms have a long history of therapeutic use in many cultures around the world. In Europe their medicinal use is documented by Dioscorides in his great work *De Materia Medica* (55AD) and by Gerrard in his influential 'Herbal' (1663)[2].

However, nowhere have their therapeutic properties been explored as comprehensively as in China and the Chinese herbal classic, the *Shen Nong Ben Cao*, dating to around 200AD, includes a number of mushrooms still in common use today, among them[3]:

- Ling Zhi (*Ganoderma lucidum* - Reishi)
- Fu Ling (*Poria cocos*)
- Bai Me Er (*Tremella fuciformis* - Snow fungus)
- Zhu Ling (*Polyporous umbellatus*)

All of these are classified in the 'Superior' category of herbs, herbs which are considered safe to take for long periods of time without side effects and of which it is said that prolonged use will 'lighten the body and confer longevity'. Indeed, *G. lucidum* is thought by many to be plant *Chi* mentioned in a number of ancient Taoist texts as a plant that brings happiness and immortality.

Over time the incorporation of mushrooms into the materia medica expanded so that in Li Shi Zhen's authoritative work, the *Ben Cao Gang Mu* (1578), 21 mushrooms are listed as having medicinal properties.

The reverence with which medicinal mushrooms, especially *G. lucidum*, are held in Chinese culture is attested to by their extensive depiction in paintings, carvings and embroidery[4].

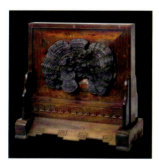

Left: Table Screen Mounted with *G. lucidum*.
THE PALACE MUSEUM, BEIJING

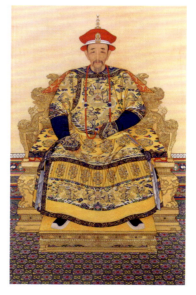

Right: Portrait of the Kangxi Emperor in Court Dress featuring *G. lucidum*-shaped cloud motif.
THE PALACE MUSEUM, BEIJING

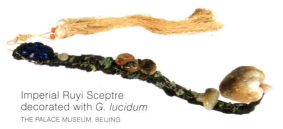

Imperial Ruyi Sceptre decorated with *G. lucidum*
THE PALACE MUSEUM, BEIJING

One of the main areas in which mushrooms have traditionally been used in the Far East is in the treatment of cancer and this led Japanese researchers in the 1960s to investigate their anti-tumour properties.

Early animal studies quickly confirmed the ability of mushroom extracts to extend survival times in a range of cancers and ultimately led to large scale clinical trials of commercial mushroom extracts.

The positive results from these trials clearly confirmed their therapeutic potential and saw their routine prescription as 'host defence potentiators', or 'biological response modifiers' (BRMs) alongside conventional cancer treatment in Japan and China[5].

Although the lack of a defined mode of action or single active chemical entity led to the failure of attempts to obtain pharmaceutical licensing in Europe and the US, the therapeutic efficacy and commercial success of these mushroom extracts has generated considerable interest in the clinical possibilities of these remarkable organisms (by 1987 sales of one, PSK or 'Krestin', from *Trametes versicolor* were over US$600 million per year and by 1993 accounted for 25% of national expenditure on anti-cancer agents in Japan[6]).

Clinical trials with PSK

CANCER TYPE	DATE	PATIENT NUMBERS	RESULT
Stomach Cancer Stage IV	1976	66	PSK doubled 2-yr survival after surgery and chemotherapy
Advanced Stomach Cancer with Metastases	1982	450	PSK doubled 5-yr survival after surgery and chemotherapy
Advanced Stomach Cancer with Metastases	1990	255	PSK extended 15-yr survival after surgery and chemotherapy
Colorectal Cancer	1990	110	PSK extended 8-yr survival and disease-free period after surgery
Lung (NSCLC) Stages I-III	1993	185	PSK extended 5-yr survival 2-4x for all stages after radiotherapy
Oesophageal	1995	158	PSK extended 5-yr survival and normalised serum factors after surgery, radiotherapy and chemotherapy
Breast Stages I, II	1995	227	PSK trend to extend 10-yr survival and disease-free period with 100% survival in patients +ve for HLA B40 antigen

After Kidd P, 2000[5].

Members of the fungal kingdom

Neither plants nor animals, mushrooms form the most visible part of the fungal kingdom, being the above ground spore-bearing fruiting bodies of 'higher fungi'. In the same way that some plants produce flowers as a means of reproduction, these fungi produce mushrooms as a means of disseminating their spores and colonizing new areas.

Although traditionally considered as closer to plants, phylogenetic research has shown that fungi are in fact more closely related to animals, sharing a common ancestor around 460 million years ago[7]. Whereas plants derive carbon from carbon dioxide in the air and energy from sunlight through photosynthesis, both fungi and animals derive carbon and energy from the enzymatic breakdown of organic matter. While animals took the evolutionary route of ingesting our food and breaking it down inside our bodies, fungi took the route of excreting enzymes into the surrounding substrate to break it down and then absorbing the smaller molecules resulting from the enzymatic hydrolysis.

Although metabolically closer to animals, structurally mushrooms are similar to plants and like them possess a rigid cell wall formed largely of long sugar molecule chains (polysaccharides – 'many sugars') joined by beta linkages and hence resistant to degradation by our digestive enzymes, which are designed to deal with the alpha-linked polysaccharides (starch) that form much of our diet.

However, unlike the cellulose in plant cell walls, which is formed by β 1→4 linked glucose molecules (adjacent glucose molecules in the chain having bonds between the 1-position carbon of one molecule and the 4-position carbon of the next), in mushrooms the main polysaccharide chain is typically β 1→3 linked with β 1→6 linked side chains, in other words a (1→3), (1→6) β-glucan.

Typical Fungal Beta-glucan. From Yanaki et al, 1983[8].

As will be discussed later, these mushroom polysaccharides have a significant impact on the immune system and the fact that they form an integral part of mushroom cell walls helps explain the broad immunomodulatory and anti-tumour activity observed in mushroom species.

Indeed, it is likely that most, if not all, of the classical mushrooms (fungi belonging to the class *Basidiomycota* that produce a spore-bearing fruiting body) contain pharmacologically active polysaccharides with polysaccharides from over 650 mushroom species already known to have anti-tumour activity[6].

In mushrooms the individual cells are joined together in long chains, or hyphae, which spread through the substrate on which the mushroom is growing, forming a tightly woven net or mycelium. The potential growth of the mycelium is limited only by the extent of the substrate and some soil growing mushrooms, such as Armillaria species (Honey Mushroom), can cover an area of over a thousand acres (the largest reported to date covers an area of 2,200 acres in eastern Oregon, USA)[9].

The fungi's reproductive organs, their spore-bearing fruiting bodies or 'mushrooms', are then produced by the mycelium in order to propagate itself and spread to new sites, often in response to exhaustion of the substrate or other environmental stress.

Rich sources of pharmacologically active compounds

In common with other fungi, which are the source of several major pharmaceutical drugs, ranging from antibiotics, such as penicillin, to statins, such as lovastatin, mushrooms produce a diverse variety of compounds with physiological activity.

In some cases these compounds are common to all mushrooms (and other fungi), ie. immunologically active beta-glucans and related polysaccharides, while others are restricted to one or a few species, ie. cyathane derivatives with the ability to stimulate production of nerve growth factor (NGF) in *Hericium erinaceus* (Lion's Mane).

The major categories of pharmacologically active compounds found in mushrooms are discussed below with species-specific compounds covered under the individual mushrooms.

Polysaccharides (beta-glucans, proteoglycans and related compounds)

Water-soluble polysaccharides and related compounds form the major class of immunologically active molecule in mushrooms and other fungi and their action on the immune system has been extensively reviewed[2,5,6].

Confusingly, several overlapping terms are in use: polysaccharides, proteoglycans (also called glycoproteins or protein-bound polysaccharides) and beta-glucans.

The term beta-glucan refers to the beta-linked glucose molecules that form the typical fungal polysaccharide. However, very few of the immunologically active polysaccharides from mushrooms are pure beta-glucans. Most are heteroglucans, containing other sugar molecules, such as galactose, xylose or mannose, as well as glucose.

Analysis of crude polysaccharide fractions from mushrooms also shows that all have some level of bound protein component (in the case of *Pleurotus citronopileatus*, the percentage of protein varies from 7-61%[6]).

Except where otherwise indicated I have therefore opted to use the broad term 'mushroom polysaccharide', including within it the beta-glucans, hetero-betaglucans and proteoglycans/glycoproteins that fall under its umbrella and are present in mushroom polysaccharide extracts.

In contrast to the relatively inexpensive commercially available beta-glucans from yeast, mushroom beta-glucans have more diverse structures and, as a consequence, higher levels of immunological activity[11]. Of the mushroom polysaccharides reported to have immunological activity 77.5% are from mushroom fruiting body, 20.8% from mycelium and 2.0% from culture filtrate (broth).

The following table illustrates the structural diversity exhibited by some immunologically active polysaccharides from common medicinal mushrooms:

MUSHROOM	IMMUNOLOGICALLY ACTIVE POLYSACCHARIDES
Agaricus brasiliensis	Various β- and α-linked glucans, Glucomannan, Riboglucan
Flammulina velutipes	Galactomannoglucan
Ganoderma lucidum	Mannogalactoglucan
Grifola frondosa	Xyloglucan, (1-6)-β-D-glucan with (1-3)-β-D-glucan side chains (MD fraction), Mannoxyloglucan, Mannogalactofucan
Hericium erinaceus	Glucoxylan, Xylan, Galactoxyloglucan, Mannoglucoxylan
Inonotus obliquus	Xylogalactoglucan
Lentinus edodes	(1-3)-β-D-glucan with (1-6)-β-D-glucosyl side chains (Lentinan), Galactoglucomannan
Trametes versicolor	Heteroglucans with α(1-4)- and β-(1-3) glycosidic linkages (with fucose in PSK and rhamnose and arabinose in PSP)
Tremella fuciformis	Glucoronoxylomannans (Tremellastin)

After Wasser SP, 2002[10]

Levels of anti-cancer activity appear to be related to degree of branching and to solubility in water, with higher solubility and a greater degree of branching being associated with higher activity (most active polysaccharides have degrees of branching between 0.20 and 0.33, ie. one side chain for every 3-5 main chain sugar units)[12].

It has also been suggested that activity may be related to molecular weight, although this may be connected to the means of administration. Higher molecular weight polysaccharides from *Lentinius edodes* (Shiitake) show higher activity when delivered by injection. However, molecular weight had no effect on the *in vitro* or orally administered activity of polysaccharides from *Tremella fuciformis* and a beta-glucan from *Agaricus brasiliensis*, which showed anti-tumour activity when delivered by injection but was found to be ineffective by oral administration, became highly effective orally after acid hydrolysis to produce shorter chains of c.10k Da size[13].

Higher levels of structure have also been investigated as possible determinants of biological activity with evidence that a triple-helical structure may be a contributing factor in the activity of some mushroom polysaccharides[10].

Proteins

As well as forming part of protein-bound polysaccharides, several mushroom proteins, including Ling Zhi-8 (LZ-8) from *Ganoderma lucidum* (Reishi) and Fve, EA-6 and Flammulin from *Flammulina velutipes* (Enokitake), have demonstrated biological activity in their own right[14-16], including:

- Immune modulation - mushroom proteins have been shown to act directly on monocytes and to effect T-cell activation

- Ribosome inactivation - several exhibit ribosome inactivating activity

- Anti-HIV - Velutin from *F. velutipes* inhibits HIV reverse transcriptase

- Anti-fungal - some have direct anti-fungal action

- Nuclease activity - a large number of proteins and peptides from mushrooms show nuclease activity

- Lectins have been isolated from many mushroom species, including *F. velutipes*, *Grifola frondosa* and *G. lucidum*[17,18]

Proteins from *F. velutipes* have also been shown to have anti-allergic properties and to increase immune response to vaccination[19].

Triterpenes

Most triterpenes are highly biologically active and those found in mushrooms are no exception. The families of ganoderic and lucidenic acids from *Ganoderma lucidum* are the best known and are responsible for many of *G. lucidum*'s unique therapeutic properties, having, among others, anti-cancer, anti-inflammatory, anti-histamine, hypotensive and sedative actions[20].

Another important terpenoid compound is betulinic acid, found in the bark of birch trees and taken up by *Inonotus obliquus* (Chaga) growing on them. Again betulinic acid demonstrates a wide range of biological activity including anti-cancer, anti-inflammatory and anti-viral properties[21].

High levels of triterpenes are also a major component responsible for the therapeutic properties of the unique Taiwanese mushroom *Antrodia camphorata*[22].

Phenols

High levels of phenolic components are found in certain mushrooms, especially *Inonotus obliquus*. Although polyphenols are known to be powerful antioxidants (the antioxidant activity of different mushrooms has been shown to be strongly correlated with their total concentrations of phenolic compounds[23]) recent publications have cast doubt on the relevance of the antioxidant properties of polyphenolic compounds such as flavonoids because of the low concentration achieved at a cellular level[24].

Instead it has been suggested that their physiological activity is a consequence of their effect on cell-signalling pathways (signal transduction pathways)[25].

Sterols

Mushrooms contain a number of sterols, principally ergosterol, with *H. erinaceus* fruiting bodies containing 381mg/100g ergosterol. In animal studies ergosterol has demonstrated activity against a number of different tumours as well as specific anti-angiogenic properties[26]. In addition, ergosterol derivatives have been reported to have anti-aging activity on a par with that of resveratrol[27].

Although ergosterol is converted into ergocalciferol, vitamin D2, on exposure to UV light, few if any supplements are produced from mushrooms exposed to sunlight and, in the absence of UV exposure, levels of vitamin D are negligible.

Chitin

The second most abundant polysaccharide in nature (after cellulose), chitin is a primary component of fungal and some bacterial cell walls, as well as the exoskeletons of insects, arachnids (spiders) and crustaceans. It is composed of beta 1,4 linked glucose units with attached acetylamine groups.

Chitin has demonstrated complex and size-dependent effects on innate and adaptive immune responses, including the ability to recruit and activate innate immune cells and induce cytokine and chemokine production via a number of cell surface receptors, including macrophage mannose receptor, TLR-2 and Dectin-1[28]. It has also demonstrated anti-bacterial and antioxidant activity and has been shown to help speed wound healing[29].

As some chitin derivatives are known to be non-toxic, non-allergenic and non-biodegradable, they are widely used in the manufacture of prostheses such as artificial skin, contact lenses and surgical stitches. However, chitin is also a common component of allergy-triggering allergens, including those in shrimp, crab and house dust mite, and may be involved in the allergic reaction to eating mushrooms seen in a small number of people (~1%)[30,31].

Enzymes

Mushrooms produce a diverse array of enzymes, including digestive enzymes (proteases, lipases, etc.) and antioxidant enzymes (laccase, catalase, superoxide dismutase (S.O.D.), etc.), and it has been suggested that the enzymatic activity of mushrooms may contribute to the therapeutic activity of fruiting body/mycelial biomass dosage forms. However, oral S.O.D. is acid-labile and has been shown to have no bio-availability, even when administered as enteric-coated capsules[32].

Tyrosinase is found in some mushrooms and has been shown to exert a genoprotective effect *in vitro*[33].

Mushroom polysaccharides - Essential nutrients for our immune system?

Polysaccharides are not the sole category of therapeutically active compound present in mushrooms but they are the most widespread and, in many but not all mushrooms, the most immunologically important, with a profound impact on the immune system mediated by a number of fungal polysaccharide-specific receptors on the surface of several important immune cell types.

The fact that so many key categories of immune cells are hard-wired to respond to the presence of fungal polysaccharides is almost certainly a consequence of our immune system having evolved under the constant challenge of fungal pathogens, the presence of which now leads to broad increase in cytotoxic immune response, not only against fungi, but also against other pathogens and cancer cells.

Fungal polysaccharide-specific receptors include:

- Dectin-1 - expressed on macrophages, monocytes, neutrophils and dendritic cells
- CR3 - expressed on neutrophils and NK Cells
- TLR - expressed on macrophages, monocytes and dendritic cells
- SIGNR1 - expressed on macrophages and dendritic cells
- LacCer - expressed on neutrophils
- Scavenger - expressed on neutrophils

Binding of fungal polysaccharides to the above receptors has been shown to trigger widespread activation of the immune system:

Immune activation induced by beta-glucans

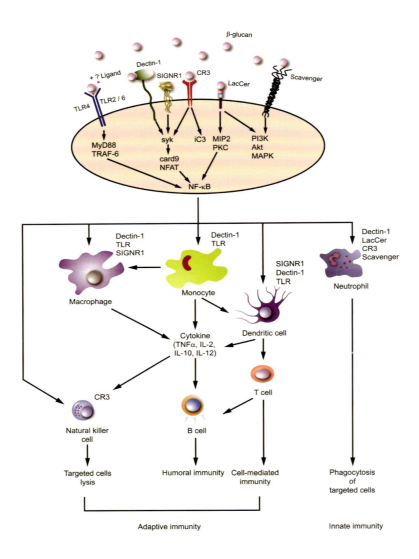

From: 'The effects of β-glucan on human immune and cancer cells'. Godfrey Chi-Fung Chan, Wing Keung Chan and Daniel Man-Yuen Sze[34].

Uptake of fungal beta-glucans and related polysaccharides appears to occur through both receptor-dependent and independent routes.

As the component sugar molecules are primarily beta linked, like cellulose, rather than alpha linked, like starch, they are not broken down by digestive enzymes and so pass intact into the small intestine. There some of them come into contact with macrophages present in the areas of lymphoid tissue in the distal small intestine called Peyer's patches or Gut Associated Lymphoid Tissue (GALT) and bind to the fungal polysaccharide-specific receptors, Dectin-1 and TLR 2/6, on their surface.

Once captured by the receptors, the polysaccharides are internalised, broken down into shorter chains and transported by the macrophages to the reticuloendothelial system where they are released to be taken up by other cells, including neutrophils, monocytes and dendritic cells, leading to activation of both the innate and specific immune systems.

As well as Dectin-1 dependent absorption of polysaccharides through GALT, it has been shown that there is Dectin-1 independent absorption through the intestinal mucosa and that polysaccharides absorbed in this way are also immunologically active, as indeed are mushroom polysaccharides such as Lentinan and Schizophyllan delivered by injection.

It has been suggested that, whereas small, soluble beta-glucans act primarily through binding to CR3, priming cells for cytotoxic activation (expressed on neutrophils and NK cells CR3 has two domains, one of which is specific for fungal polysaccharides and binding to which greatly enhances the ability of the cells to effectively target and destroy antibody-coated cancer cells and other pathogens), larger polysaccharide molecules are able to cross-link membrane CR3 of neutrophils and monocytes, triggering respiratory bursts, degranulation and cytokine release[35].

The uptake and subsequent actions of beta-glucans on immune cells

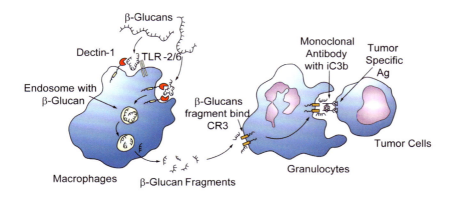

From: 'The effects of β-glucan on human immune and cancer cells'. Godfrey Chi-Fung Chan, Wing Keung Chan and Daniel Man-Yuen Sze[34].

Not only does binding of fungal polysaccharides to the aforementioned receptors lead to a significant increase in cytotoxic ability, it also initiates widespread activation of the immune system (see below), with the term 'biological response modifier' used to reflect the ability to modify, or modulate, immune response.

Immune responses to fungal polysaccharides

- Increased Antibody Production
- Increased Lymphocyte Activating Factor (IL-1) Production
- Increased Tumour Necrosis Factor Production
- Increased Colony Stimulating Factor Production
- Increased Complement C3 Production
- Increased IFN-γ Production
- Increased IL-2 Production
- Reduction in the level of IL-2 needed to produce a cytotoxic response
- Th1 Activation
- Macrophage Activation
- Neutrophil Activation
- Natural Killer Cell Activation
- Cytotoxic T-cell Activation
- Lymphokine Activated Killer Cell Proliferation
- Enhanced maturation and tumour infiltration of Dendritic Cells
- Th2 Suppression
- Reduced IL-4 Production
- Inhibition of Prostaglandin Synthesis
- Inhibition of Delayed type Hypersensitivity

Of particular importance for the impact of medicinal mushrooms on many chronic health disorders is the ability of mushroom polysaccharides to promote a shift in the pattern of immune response in chronic conditions such as cancer, auto-immune and allergic conditions from a pro-inflammatory, Th2 dominant one to a cytotoxic, Th1 dominant one with increases in Th1 cytokines such as IL-2 and IFN-γ and decreases in Th2 cytokines such as IL-4.

Pharmacokinetics of Mushroom Polysaccharides

Studies with radio-labelled PSK showed it to be partially decomposed to smaller molecules in the digestive tract with the full molecular spectrum of of radio-labelled PSK absorbed within 24 hrs following oral administration in mice. Peak plasma levels of low molecular weight substances occur at 0.5-1 hr in rats and 1-2 hr in rabbits, while PSK size molecules appear in the serum after 4, 10 and 24hr[32].

Radio-labelled PSK or its metabolites are detected in the intestinal tract, bone marrow, salivary glands, thymus, adrenal glands, brain, liver, spleen, pancreas and tumour tissue in sarcoma-bearing mice, with activity high for longest in the liver and bone marrow.

86% of PSK is excreted within 24hr (~70% excreted in expired air, 20% in faeces, 10% in urine and 0.8% in bile).

Th1-Th2, Mushroom Polysaccharides and Immune Balance

The terms Th1 and Th2 refer to two major populations of T-helper cells, a subset of lymphocytes (a type of white blood cell) that plays an important role in establishing and maximising the capabilities of the immune system. They are involved respectively in promoting cellular (cytotoxic) and humoral (pro-inflammatory) immune responses[36].

The balance between a Th1 and a Th2-mediated immune response appears to play an important role in immune regulation with a number of chronic disease states, including cancer, allergies and asthma, exhibiting elevated levels of the cytokines (chemical messengers) characteristic of a Th2 dominant immune response.

In a balanced state the immune system is able to maintain an equilibrium between Th1 and Th2 mediated immune responses but it appears that in these conditions a shift has taken place with the immune system becoming locked into a Th2 dominant pattern with increased levels of inflammation, metabolic activity and, in the case of cancer, angiogenesis (blood vessel formation), as well as reduced cytotoxic activity. Stress, elevated cortisol levels and exposure to organic pesticides have all been suggested as possible causes.

Supplementation with mushroom polysaccharides shows a clear shift in immune balance towards Th1 dominance with increased production of Th1 cytokines such as IL-2 and IFN-γ and suppression of Th2 cytokine production. As such it offers a valuable therapeutic tool for addressing a Th1→Th2 shift in conditions such as those mentioned above.

The concept of a Th1→Th2 shift in immune balance finds parallels in the traditional Chinese medical concept of Retained Pathogenic Factor/Latent Heat, which describes many of the signs and symptoms characteristic of a Th2 dominant immune state, including fatigue, reduced resistance to infection, depression and chronic low-grade inflammation and medicinal mushrooms can likewise play an important role in treatment strategies.

Understanding Mushroom Products

As well as having a large number of mushrooms with similar properties to choose from, the therapist is faced with an often bewildering variety of product forms produced through different growing and manufacturing processes.

Whereas traditionally only the fruiting body, or in some cases the sclerotium (underground hyphal mass - ie. *Polyporus umbellatus* and *Poria cocos*) or conk (sterile fungal growth on the trunk of the tree - ie. *Inonotus obliquus* - Chaga), was harvested and either been consumed whole in food, as with *Lentinus edodes* (Shiitake) and *Grifola frondosa* (Maitake), or as teas made from aqueous decoctions of the fruiting body, as with *Ganoderma lucidum* (Reishi) and *I. obliquus*, nowadays many commercial mushroom products are produced from the mycelium of the mushroom grown either by liquid state fermentation or solid state fermentation (biomass).

The following overview summarizes the features of the different dosage forms available.

Fruiting Body/Conk/Sclerotium

The traditional dosage form of medicinal mushrooms, the fruiting body typically contains a higher level and number of different polysaccharides than the mycelium or culture broth with a beta-glucan content of 41% reported for *G. lucidum* fruiting body by Stamets[7]. A higher level of water soluble polysaccharides is also reported in the conk or sclerotium, with the conk of *I. obliquus* having 176.5g/kg (dry weight) soluble polysaccharides and the mycelium 53.9g/kg (dry weight)[6].

Research into beta-glucans from *L. edodes* and *G. frondosa* showed an increase in concentration with fruiting body growth until an optimum size was reached (approx. 17g for *L. edodes* and 180g for *G. frondosa*), after which levels declined[37].

In addition, concentrations of components such as triterpenes (*G. lucidum*) and other phenolic compounds (*I. obliquus*) tend to be higher in the fruiting body, where their bitter taste and natural anti-microbial properties act to discourage unwanted predators. Data from *Antrodia camphorata* suggests the level of triterpenes in the mycelium is 40% of that in the fruiting body and for many biomass products the relative discrepancy is likely to be larger owing to the presence of residual substrate in the biomass (less than 100% of the biomass is mycelium). For this reason *G. lucidum* biomass products tend to lack the characteristic bitter flavour of the triterpenes found largely in the fruiting body.

Extracts

For mushrooms where triterpenoid and other phenolic components are therapeutically important, i.e. *A. camphorata, G. lucidum, I. obliquus*, products derived from the fruiting body/conk are usual with, given their indigestible nature, extracts often used in agreement with traditional practice.

Extracts are also used to deliver high concentrations of polysaccharides or other active components. They are usually made from either the fruiting body or the mycelium through one of two main methods:

- Aqueous extraction (traditional teas/decoctions) gives high polysaccharide concentrations but low levels of poorly water-soluble triterpenes. Crude polysaccharide extracts typically have around 30% polysaccharides with further purification possible.
- Ethanolic (alcohol) extraction (traditional tinctures) extracts more triterpenes but fewer polysaccharides (ethanol precipitates the polysaccharides out of solution).

As well as offering higher concentrations of polysaccharides and other clinically important compounds, extracts may be preferred in cases of gut dysbiosis, from antibiotic use or otherwise, with resultant impaired ability to break down whole mushroom or biomass products (also in cases of colostomy).

For some mushrooms such as *G. lucidum*, aqueous extracts and ethanolic extracts can be combined to deliver high concentrations of both polysaccharides and triterpenes. Some practitioners such as Nanba have also reported good results from combining high concentration polysaccharide (beta-glucan) extracts with whole mushroom fruiting body or biomass[38].

Spores

The fruiting body exists to spread the spores of the mushroom and some products use the spores themselves. Together with polysaccharides, triterpenes and sterols the spores are rich in fatty acids, which have been implicated in their therapeutic action[39-41]. However, studies comparing the immunological activity of *G. lucidum* spores and unpurified fruiting body show little difference[42].

Mycelium (liquid/submerged fermentation)

Liquid fermentation is the same technology used in the pharmaceutical industry to produce antibiotics and also to produce other industrial products such as fungal enzymes.

The mushroom mycelium is cultured in a closed vessel with a liquid substrate containing all the essential nutrients for growth and growth parameters such as nutrient composition and temperature carefully controlled to optimise concentration of the desired components.

Because the substrate is a liquid the mycelium can easily be harvested and then either used as a therapeutic component itself or in most cases further processed to yield various extracts (eg. PSK and Lentinan). In addition, the extracellular metabolites secreted into the growth medium (broth) may also be harvested for their therapeutic properties (eg. Schizophyllan, an extra-cellular polysaccharide from *Schizophyllum commune*).

Mycelial Biomass (solid state fermentation)

In solid state fermentation (often referred to as biomass production) the mushroom culture is inoculated into a sterile, grain-based substrate, usually brown rice, and left to fully colonize the substrate. At the point at which it has exhausted the capacity of the substrate to support further growth and is about to produce fruiting bodies (primordia stage) the resultant mass of mycelium and residual substrate is dried and granulated to make a powder, which is then usually tabletted or encapsulated.

As well as mushroom mycelium and some residual grain, biomass products contain the full range of metabolites excreted into the substrate by the mycelium (especially antibiotics and exopolysaccharides), together with a wide variety of enzymes, including digestive enzymes (proteases, lipases etc.) and antioxidant enzymes (laccase, catalase and superoxide dismutase). They also contain substrate breakdown products such as arabinoxylans with therapeutic properties in their own right. Indeed, in supplements such as Biobran™, also known as MGN-3™ (shiitake digested rice bran) and Avemar™ (yeast digested wheatgerm) the enzymatically transformed substrate itself is seen as the therapeutic entity.

Stamets reports crude arabinoxylane content of mushroom mycelial biomass cultivated on short grain brown rice by his company, Fungi Perfecti, as ranging from 7.8% in *Agaricus brasiliensis* to 24% in *Cordyceps sinensis*.

While mushroom biomass products contain a wide range of bioactive molecules, levels of the key immunomodulating beta-glucans and related heteropolysaccharides are low. Stamets reports beta-glucan levels in the above form of biomass ranging from 1.23% in *Hericium erinaceus* to 2.96% in *I. obliquus* with *A. brasiliensis* 1.83%, *G. frondosa* 2.51% and *G. lucidum* 2.19%. At the same time he reports the beta-glucan content in mushroom fruiting bodies as varying from 8.9% in *A. brasiliensis* to 14.5% in *G. frondosa* and 41% in *G. lucidum*[7].

These figures for beta-glucan concentrations in biomass products are consistent with those obtained by the author on biomass samples from other manufacturers.

Combination Products

There is evidence that combinations of mushrooms can have a greater effect on the immune system of both humans and mice than single mushrooms.

Ghoneum et al[43] report synergistic action between different mushrooms and, in a 2002 paper, Sawai et al report greater immunological activity with higher levels of macrophage activation and INF-y induction by a mixture of mushroom polysaccharide extracts than by the single extracts[44]. Stamets also reports a blend of seven mushrooms (biomass) as having enhanced NK cell activation in human spleen cells when compared to the individual mushrooms[45].

Prescribing Medicinal Mushrooms

Prescribing medicinal mushrooms is not an exact science. Dosage depends on the condition and the individual being treated, as well as the product format being prescribed, and is discussed under the individual mushrooms and under the different clinical conditions, including at the end of the section on Medicinal Mushrooms in Cancer Therapy.

Although many of the medicinal mushrooms are also foods, for therapeutic purposes it is preferable to take them away from food to avoid interfering with their absorption. However, it can be appropriate to give together with juices, smoothies or pureed fruit to assist with swallowing, depending on the format and the individual.

While it is common to split the prescribed dose into two, with one taken a.m. and one p.m., it can be split into three if that is easier, especially for higher doses, or taken in a single dose if two is not possible. In all cases it is beneficial to take with 1-2 glasses of water.

Are there any side effects?

Exhaustive analysis of data from several large scale clinical trials with mushroom polysaccharides confirms that side effects from mushroom supplements are minimal. In a study of 469 patients taking Lentinan only 32 reported any adverse reaction, none serious (most common were rash/redness, chest oppression and nausea), and a review in the Lancet of a well designed trial investigating the benefit of PSK for gastric cancer concluded that no toxic effects could be observed 'even after meticulous review of all the patient records'[5].

Clinically some change in bowel habit is seen in a few patients, especially at higher dosages but this is usually transient, lasting no more than 2-3 days.

Supplementation with medicinal mushrooms should of course be avoided in individuals with a history of confirmed or suspected mushroom allergy.

Can I use mushroom supplements for patients with candidiasis or other fungal conditions?

Yes! The common myth that eating mushrooms will in some way facilitate the growth of candida or other fungal conditions is unsupported by clinical experience or research evidence.

Not only are mushrooms very low in the sugars that are considered by some to promote candidal growth but they also strengthen the body's immune response to all fungi and in some cases contain compounds with direct anti-fungal activity (see Candidiasis for a more detailed discussion).

But aren't mushrooms considered Damp in traditional Chinese medicine (TCM)?

No. While some mushrooms are considered to nourish Yin energy (ie. *Tremella fuciformis* - Bai Mu Er), none of them are considered to increase pathogenic Damp. Indeed for two of them (*Polyporus umbellatus* - Zhu Ling and *Poria cocos* - Fu Ling) the main use in TCM is as diuretics to Drain Damp and clinically mushrooms can be very beneficial in the treatment of conditions that are considered Damp in TCM, such as candidiasis.

Appendix I lists the TCM qualities of the main medicinal mushrooms.

Can mushrooms be taken alongside conventional treatment?

In many cases the mushrooms used medicinally are also foodstuffs and in the vast majority of cases there are no reported interactions with prescription medication. Indeed mushroom extracts are routinely prescribed alongside prescription drugs, especially chemotherapeutic agents, in China and Japan (see Medicinal Mushrooms in Cancer Therapy for a more detailed discussion of this area).

There is also evidence from research on the combination of Maitake D-fraction (10mg/kg/day) and vancomycin (10mg/kg/day) in the treatment of methicillin-resistant *Staphylococcus aureus* (MRSA) in mice that mushroom polysaccharides can improve the effectiveness of antibiotics with an increased survival rate in mice given both the antibiotic and the polysaccharide extract[46].

One report of an HIV patient being treated with *Trametes versicolor* biomass and Chinese herbs indicated deterioration of immune parameters during administration of a broad spectrum antibiotic and it may be that an intact intestinal flora is important for the efficacy of biomass products with the bacteria in the intestines helping to break them down and increase their bioavailability[47].

Specific cautions are noted in the sections on the individual mushrooms.

Can pregnant or breastfeeding women take medicinal mushrooms?

With the exception of *Auricularia auricula*, tests with commercial mushroom products show no adverse affect on male or female fertility, foetal abnormality, penetration into the foetus or excretion in breast milk, blood coagulation or arthritis from polysaccharide-based products. Neither do they possess teratogenic or genotoxic properties[48].

Anti-fertility action has been reported for *A. auricula* polysaccharides and for this reason neither *A. auricula* or *T. fuciformis*, whose polysaccharides have a similar structure, are recommended for use during pregnancy or if pregnancy is planned.[49]

REFERENCES

1. Medicinal mushroom science: history, current status, future trends and unsolved problems. Wasser S.P. Int J Med Mushr. 2010;12(1):1-16
2. Medicinal mushrooms - An Exploration of Tradition, Healing and Culture. Hobbs C. 1986. Pub. Botanica Press, Williams. p.7-10
3. ibid. p.20-26
4. Reishi Mushroom - Herb of Spiritual Potency and Medical Wonder. Willard T. 1990 Sylvan Press. Issaquah
5. The use of mushroom glucans and proteoglycans in cancer treatment. Kidd P. Alt Med J. 2000;5(1):4-27
6. Higher Basidiomycota as a source of antitumour and immuno-stimulating polysaccharides (Review). Reshetnikov S.V, Tan K.K. Int J Med Mushr. 2001;3(4):361-394
7. Potentiation of cell-mediated host defense using fruitbodies and mycelia of medicinal mushrooms. Stamets P. Int J Med Mushr. 2003;5:179-191
8. Correlation between the antitumour activity of a polysaccharide schizophyllan and its triple-helical conformation in dilute aqueous solution. Yanaki T, Ito W, Tabata K, Kojima T, Norisuye T, Takano N, Fujita H. Biophys Chem. 1983; 17(4):337-42

9. Medicinal mushrooms: their therapeutic properties and current medical usage with special emphasis on cancer treatments. Smith J, Rowan N, Sullivan R. May 2002. Cancer Research UK. p.17
10. Medicinal mushrooms as a source of antitumour and immuno-modulating polysaccharides. Wasser S.P. Appl. Environ Microbiol. 2002;60:258-274
11. Evaluation of widely consumed botanicals as immunological adjuvants. Ragupathi G, Yeung K.S, Leung P.C, Lee M, Lau C.B, Vickers A, Hood C, Deng G, Cheung N.K, Cassileth B, Livingston P. Vaccine. 2008;26(37):4860-5
12. Medicinal mushrooms: their therapeutic properties and current medical usage with special emphasis on cancer treatments. Smith J, Rowan N, Sullivan R. May 2002. Cancer Research UK. p.101
13. Peroral effect on tumour progression of soluble beta 1-6 glucans prepared by acid treatment from *Agaricus blazei*. Murr. Fujiyama Y, Yamomoto H, Noji M, Suzuki I. Int J Med Mush 2000;2:43-49
14. Mushroom proteins related to host defense. Ng T.B. Int J Med Mush. 2005;7(1,2):221-236
15. Immunomodulatory capacity of fungal proteins on the cytokine production of human peripheral blood mononuclear cells. Jeurink P.V, Noguera C.L, Savelkoul H.F, Wichers H.J. Int Immuno-pharmacol. 2008;8(8):1124-33
16. Polysaccharides PS-G and protein LZ-8 from Reishi (*Ganoderma lucidum*) exhibit diverse functions in regulating murine macrophages and T lymphocytes. Yeh C.H, Chen H.C, Yang J.J, Chuang W.I, Sheu F. J Agric Food Chem. 2010;58(15):8535-44
17. Lectins of higher fungi (Macromycetes)—their occurrence, physiological role, and biological activity. Konska G. Int J Med Mush. 2006;8(1):19-30
18. Comparative study of lectin activity of higher Basidiomycetes. Nona A., Mikiashvili N.A, Elisashvili V, Wasser S.P, Nevo E. Int J Med Mush. 2006;8(1):31-38
19. Coadministration of the fungal immunomodulatory protein FIP-Fve and a tumour-associated antigen enhanced antitumour immunity. Ding Y, Seow S.V, Huang C.H, Liew L.M, Lim Y.C, Kuo I.C, Chua K.Y. Immunology. 2009;128(1Sup):881-94
20. Biomedical triterpenoids of *Ganoderma lucidum* (Curt.: Fr.) P. Karst. (Aphyllophoromycetideae). Kim H.W, Kim B.K, Int J Med Mushr. 1999;1:121-13817
21. Betulinic acid, a natural compound with potent anticancer effects. Mullauer F.B, Kessler J.H, Medema J.P. Anticancer Drugs. 2010;21(3):215-27. 2010;24(1):90-114
22. Review of pharmacological effects of *Antrodia camphorata* and its bioactive compounds. Geethangili M, Tzeng Y.M. Evid Based Complement Alternat Med. 2009
23. Antioxidant properties of several medicinal mushrooms. Mau JL, Lin HC, Chen CC.J Agric Food Chem. 2002 Oct 9; 50(21):6072-7
24. Flavonoids: antioxidants or signalling molecules?. Williams R.J, Spencer J.P, Rice-Evans C. Free Radical Biology & Medicine. 2004;36(7):838–49
25. Regulation of cellular signals from nutritional molecules: a specific role for phytochemicals, beyond antioxidant activity. Virgili F, Marino M. Free Radical Biology & Medicine. 2008;45(9):1205–16
26. Isolation of an antitumour compound (Ergosterol) from *Agaricus blazei* Murill and its mechanism of action. Takaku T, Kimura Y, Okuda H. J Nutr. 2001;131:1409–1413
27. Ganodermasides A and B, two novel anti-aging ergosterols from spores of a medicinal mushroom *Ganoderma lucidum* on yeast via UTH1 gene. Weng Y, Xiang L, Matsuura A, Zhang Y, Huang Q, Qi J. Bioorg Med Chem. 2010;18(3):999-1002
28. Chitin Regulation of Immune Responses: An Old Molecule With New Roles. Lee CG, Da Silva CA, Lee JY, Hartl D, Elias JA. Curr Opin Immunol. 2008; 20(6):684–689
29. Fungal chitin in medicine:prospects for its application. Burdyukova L.I, Gorovoj L.F. Int J Med Mush. 2001;3(2-3):126-127
30. Mushroom allergy. Koivikko A, Savolainen J. Allergy. 1988 Jan;43(1): 1-10
31. Chitin induces accumulation in tissue of innate immune cells associated with allergy. Nature. 2007;447;(7140):92–96
32. Herb-Drug Interactions in Oncology. Cassileth BR, Yeung KS, Gubili J. Memorial Sloan-Kettering Cancer Center. 2010 People's Medical Publishing House, Shelton
33. Role of tyrosinase in the genoprotective effect of the edible mushroom, *Agaricus bisporus*. Shi Y.L, Benzie I.F.F, Buswell J.A. Life Sciences 2002;70(14):1595-1608
34. The effects of β-glucan on human immune and cancer cells. Godfrey Chi-Fung Chan, Wing Keung Chan and Daniel Man-Yuen Sze31. Journal of Hematology & Oncology 2009, 2:25
35. Therapeutic intervention with complement and beta-glucan in cancer. Ross GD, Vetvicka V, Yan J, Xia Y, Vetvickova J. Immunopharmacology. 1999;42:61-74
36. TH1/Th2 Balance: the hypothesis, its limitations and implications for health and disease. Kidd P. Alt Med Rev. 2003;8(3):223-246
37. Changes in immunomodulating activities and content of antitumour polysaccharides during the growth of two medicinal mushrooms, *Lentinus edodes* (Berk.) Sing, and *Grifola frondosa* (Dicks.: Fr.) S. F. Gray. Minato K.I, Mizuno M, Kawakami S, Tatsuoka S, Denpo Y, Tokimoto K, Tsuchida H. Int J Med Mush. 2001;3(1):1-8
38. Maitake extracts and their therapeutic potential - A review. Mayell M. Alt Med Rev, 2001;6(1)
39. Antitumour activity of the sporoderm-broken germinating spores of *Ganoderma lucidum*. Liu X, Yuan J.P, Chung C.K, Chen X.J. Cancer Lett. 2002;182(2):155-61
40. Sterols and triterpenoids from the spores of *Ganoderma lucidum*. Zhang C.R, Yang S.P, Yue J.M. Nat Prod Res. 2008;22(13):1137-42
41. Chemical constituents of the spores of *Ganoderma lucidum*. Zhang X.Q, Pang G.L, Cheng Y, Wang Y, Ye W.C. Zhong Yao Cai. 2008;31(1):41-4
42. Comparative studies on the immunomodulatory and antitumour activities of the different parts of fruiting body of *Ganoderma lucidum* and *Ganoderma* spores. Yue G.G, Fung K.P, Leung P.C, Lau C.B. Phytother Res. 2008;22(10):1282-91
43. Immunomodulatory and anticancer effects of active hemicellulose compound (AHCC). Ghoneum M, Wimbley M, Salem F, McKlain A, Attalah N, Gill G. Int J Immunotherapy. 1995;1,1:23-28
44. Extraction of conformationally stable (1-6)-branched (1-3)-β-glucans from premixed edible mushroom powders by cold-alkaline solution. Sawai, M., Adachi, Y., Kanai, M., Matsui, S. and Yadomae, T. Int J Med Mushr. 2002;4:3
45. Potentiation of cell-mediated host defense using fruitbodies and mycelia of medicinal mushrooms. P.Stamets. Int J Med Mushr. 2003;5:179-191
46. Addition of Maitake D-fraction reduces the effective dosage of vancomycin for the treatment of Listeria-infected mice. Reese T.A, Liang H, Tager A.M, Luster A.D, Van Rooijen N, Voehringer D, Locksley R.M, Kodama N, Yamada M, Nanba H. Jpn J Pharmacol. 2001;87(4):327-32
47. The clinical use of *Coriolus versicolor* supplementation in HIV+ patients and the impact on CD4 count and viral load. Pfeiffer M. 3rd International Symposium on Mushroom Nutrition. Milan 2001
48. Medicinal mushrooms: their therapeutic properties and current medical usage with special emphasis on cancer treatments. Smith J, Rowan N, Sullivan R. May 2002. Cancer Research UK. p.166-168
49. Anti-fertility action of *Auricularia auricula* polysaccharide. He B. Chen Q. Zhongguo Yaoke Daxue Xuebao. 1991;22:48-49

Medicinal Mushrooms

To date around 14,000 species of mushroom have been described, although it is believed that the actual number is ten times as large. Of these it has been estimated that 5% may be therapeutically useful.

Any selection of medicinal mushrooms is therefore inevitably going to be a partial one but I have tried to include those mushrooms with significant therapeutic potential that is supported by traditional use and clinical research.

Agaricus Brasiliensis
(Agaricus blazei/Agaricus subrufescens)

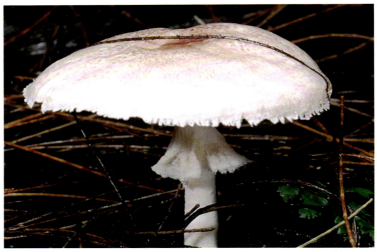

© 2010 Taylor F. Lockwood

Japanese name
Himematsutake

Portuguese name
Cogumela del sol

English name
Royal/Sun Agaric

Although commonly known as *A. blazei* Murrill (ABM), after a mushroom discovered in 1945 by the mycologist William A. Murrill growing on the lawn of his friend R.W. Blaze in Florida, the mushroom used therapeutically can be traced to spores and samples sent to Japan from the Piedade region of Brazil by a farmer of Japanese descent in 1965. It is now believed that the two are in fact different species with the name *Agaricus brasiliensis* proposed for the Brazilian mushroom[1]. It has also been suggested that *A. blazei* is the same mushroom first identified by Charles Horton Peck in 1893 and called *A. subrufescens*[2].

Although one of the newest medicinal mushrooms, *A. brasiliensis* is rapidly becoming one of the most popular. Reported in a recent survey to be taken by 31% of urological cancer patients in Japan[3], with the fastest growing US sales of any medicinal mushroom[4] and one of the three most popular medicinal mushrooms in Taiwan, this relative of the common button mushroom, *A. bisporus*, exhibits broad clinical activity[5].

Its polysaccharides include several immunologically active low molecular weight fractions, while an α-1,6 and α-1,4 glucan complex, several polysaccharide-protein complexes, a glucomannan with a main chain of beta 1,2 linked mannopyranosyle residues and a heteropolysaccharide composed mainly of glucose, arabinose and mannose all show anti-tumour activity[6-17]. Interestingly there appears to be an increase in structural diversity of its polysaccharides with maturation of the fruiting body[18].

A. brasiliensis also contains high levels of lipids, including linoleic acid, oleic acid, stearic acid and ergosterol[19].

CANCER - *A. brasiliensis* polysaccharide extracts show strong *in vitro* and *in vivo* activity against a range of cancer cell lines, including lung and ovarian cancer, and *in vivo* studies show positive results for Ehrlich ascites cancer, Sarcoma 180, human ovarian cancer and mouse lung cancer cell lines, as well as synergistic benefits with chemotherapy and radiotherapy[20].

In a rat cachexia model *A. brasiliensis* extracts, as well as powdered fruiting body, significantly reduced tumour size and promoted gain in body weight with reduction in AST levels and increased glycemia[21], while an *in vivo* study using severely immunodeficient mice found *A. brasiliensis* polysaccharides to directly inhibit the growth of prostate cancer cells via an apoptotic pathway and to suppress prostate tumour growth via anti-proliferative and anti-angiogenic mechanisms with the greatest activity found in the broth fraction (compounds extracted from the liquid growth medium on which the mycelium was grown) rather than the mushroom itself[22].

A 2008 study reported significant increases in the NK cell activity of human volunteers with *A. brasiliensis* polysaccharide extract at a dose of 3g/day compared to placebo,[23] while Ahn reports increased NK-cell activity and reduced chemotherapy related side effects (appetite loss, alopecia, emotional stability, and general weakness) from *A. brasiliensis* polysaccharide extract in one hundred cervical, ovarian, and endometrial cancer patients treated either with carboplatin plus VP16 (etoposide) or with carboplatin plus taxol[24].

In two small Chinese clinical studies, a dose of 20g *A. brasiliensis* fruiting body, twice a day taken as a tea (hot water extract), was reported to improve hematopoietic parameters and treatment outcomes in patients receiving chemotherapy for acute non-lymphocytic leukaemia in one study and improvement in immune status, hematopoietic parameters and quality of life measures in late stage alimentary tract tumours in another[25,26].

The closely related *A. bisporus* shows *in vitro* anti-aromatase activity, with conjugated linoleic acid identified as the main active component, and Mizuno reports positive clinical results with *A. brasiliensis* in a number of mainly breast cancer patients but at unspecified dosage[27-29].

Although most of the published research strongly supports the use of *A. brasiliensis* in cancer therapy, two studies studies looking at the protective properties of *A. brasiliensis* have been published with negative outcomes (in one *A. brasiliensis* given at 5% of diet did not have a suppressive effect on colon carcinogenesis in rats exposed to dimethylhydrazine and in another an aqueous extract did not affect the development of liver cancer induced by diethylnitrosamine) and it appears that there may be significant variation in activity between different extracts, as well as between different strains[30-33].

DIABETES - To date little clinical data has been published, although a 2008 study reported decreases in cholesterol and glucose levels, together with increased natural killer cell activity at a dose of 3g/day polysaccharide extract[23].

ALLERGIES - As potent immune modulators mushroom polysaccharides can reduce the level of Th2 mediated allergic reactions and *A. brasiliensis* is no exception with Andosan, a proprietary combination of polysaccharide extracts from *A. brasiliensis* (82%), *H. erinaceus* (15%) and *G. frondosa* (3%), causing a shift towards a Th1 cytokine profile with consequent reduced risk of allergies and *in vitro* inhibition of histamine release from mast cells[34].

HEPATOPROTECTIVE - There is evidence from a number of small clinical studies indicating possible application of *A. brasiliensis* in the treatment of chronic hepatitis. In one study 1500mg of polysaccharide extract produced significant reductions in liver enzymes in a small number of hepatitis B patients over a 12 month period (AST reduced from 246 to 61 and ALT from 151 to 46)[35]. In another *A. brasiliensis* extract reduced GTP in 80% of 20 patients with hepatitis C[36]. Wang et al also reported wide-ranging benefits in patients with chronic Hepatitis B at a dose of 20g fruiting body twice a day over a 3 month period, including reduction in abdominal distension, fatigue and hepatodynia, together with increased retraction of the liver and spleen[37].

CLINICAL SUMMARY

Main Therapeutic Application - *Cancer*

Key Component - *Polysaccharides*

Dose - *3g/day polysaccharide extract has been used in clinical trials but the high activity of the culture broth also supports the use of biomass or of biomass/polysaccharide extract combinations*

Caution - *One report has suggested a possible connection between consumption of an A. brasiliensis extract and three cases of hepatic dysfunction in cancer patients, although the authors state that several other causative factors cannot be completely ruled out[38]. Cheilitis due to an A. brasiliensis extract has also been reported[39].*

REFERENCES

1. Nutritional and chemical composition of culinary-medicinal Royal Sun Agaricus (the Himematsutake mushroom) *Agaricus brasiliensis* S. Wasser et al. (Agaricomycetideae). Menezes M.C, Eira A.F, Silva G.F, Martins O.A, Meira D.R, Caramori C.A. Int J Med Mushr. 2008;10(2):189-194

2. *Agaricus subrufescens*, a cultivated edible and medicinal mushroom, and its synonyms. Kerrigan R.W. Mycologia. 2005;97(1):12-24

3. Use of complementary and alternative medicine by patients with urologic cancer: a prospective study at a single Japanese institution. Yoshinura W, Ueda N, Ichioka K, Matsui Y, Terai A, Arai Y. Support Care Cancer. 2005;13:685-90

4. Uncloaking the mysteries of medicinal mushrooms: the U.S. medicinal mushroom market continues to grow and evolve rapidly but its size still pales in comparison to the rest of the world. Adams C. Nutraceuticals World. October 01, 2008

5. The medicinal mushroom *Agaricus blazei* Murrill: Review of literature and Pharmaco-toxicological problems. Firenzuoli F, Gori L, Lombardo G. Evid Based Complement Alternat Med. 2008;5(1):3-15

6. Characterization of chemical composition of *Agaricus brasiliensis* polysaccharides and its effect on myocardial SOD activity, MDA and caspase-3 level in ischemia-reperfusion rats. Zhang S, He B, Ge J, Zhai C, Liu X, Liu P. Int J Biol Macromol.2010;46(3):363-6

7. Structural characterization of a water-soluble β-d-glucan from fruiting bodies of *Agaricus blazei* Murrill. Dong Q, Yao J, Yang X.T and Fang J.N. Carbohyd. Res. 2007;337:1417–1421

8. Antitumour beta-glucan from the cultured fruit body of *Agaricus blazei*. Ohno N, Furukawa N, and Miura N. Biol Pharm Bull. 2004;24:820–828

9. Tumour-specific cytocidal and immunopotentiating effects of relatively low molecular weight products derived from the basidiomycete *Agaricus blazei* Murrill. Fujimiya Y, Suzuki Y, Katakura R, and Ebina T. Anticancer Res. 1999;19:113–118

10. Immunostimulatory activities of a low molecular weight antitumoural polysaccharide isolated from *Agaricus blazei* Murill (LMPAB) in Sarcoma 180 ascitic tumour-bearing mice. Niu Y.C, Liu J.C, Zhao X.M, Su F.Q, Cui H.X. Pharmazie. 2009;64(7):472-6

11. Isolation and characterization of polysaccharides from *Agaricus blazei* Murrill. Gonzaga M.L.C, Ricardo N.M.P.S, Heatley F, and Soares S.A. Carbohyd. Polym. 2005;60:43–49

12. Antitumour effect of a peptide-glucan preparation extracted from *Agaricus blazei* in a double-grafted tumour system in mice. Ebina T, and Fujimiya Y. Biotherapy. 1998;11:259–265

13. Fractionation and antitumour activity of the water-insoluble residue of *Agaricus blazei* fruiting bodies. Kawagishi H, Inagaki R, Kanao T, Mizuno T, Shimura K, Ito H, Hagiwar T, and NakamuraT. Carbohyd. Res. 1989;186:267–273

14. Oral administration of *Agaricus brasiliensis* S. Wasser et al. (Agarico-mycetideae) extract downregulates serum immunoglobulin E levels by enhancing Th1 response. Morimoto T, Michihiro T.M, Masashi M.M. Int J Med Mushr 2008;10(1):30

15. An extract based on the medicinal mushroom *Agaricus blazei* Murill stimulates monocyte-derived dendritic cells to cytokine and chemokine production *in vitro*. Førland D.T, Johnson E, Tryggestad A.M, Lyberg T, Hetland G. Cytokine. 2010 Mar;49 (3):245-50

16. Effect of an extract based on the medicinal mushroom *Agaricus blazei* murill on release of cytokines, chemokines and leukocyte growth factors in human blood *ex-vivo* and *in vivo*. Johnson E, Førland D.T, Saetre L, Bernardshaw S.V, Lyberg T, Hetland G, Scand J. Immunol. 2009;69(3):242-50

17. Peroral effect on tumour progression of soluble beta 1-6 glucans prepared by acid treatment from *Agaricus blazei* Murr. Fujiyama Y, Yamomoto H, Noji M, Suzuki I. Int J Med Mush 2000;2:43-4912

18. Structural characterization of beta-glucans of *Agaricus brasiliensis* in different stages of fruiting body maturity and their use in nutraceutical products. Camelini C.M, Maraschin M, de Mendonça M.M, Zucco C, Ferreira A.G, Tavares L.A. Biotechnol Lett. 2005;27(17):1295-9

19. Isolation of an antitumour compound (Ergosterol) from *Agaricus blazei* Murill and its mechanism of action. Takaku T, Kimura Y, Okuda H.J. Nutr. 2001;131:1409–1413

20. Suppressing effects of daily oral supplementation of beta-glucan extracted from *Agaricus blazei* Murill on spontaneous and peritoneal disseminated metastasis in mouse model. Kobayashi H, Yoshida R, Kanada Y, Fukuda Y, Yagyu T, Inagaki K, Kondo T, Kurita N, Suzuki M, Kanayama N, Terao J. J Cancer Res Clin Oncol. 2005;131(8):527-38

21. Effects of *Agaricus brasiliensis* mushroom in Walker-256 tumour-bearing rats. Jumes F.M, Lugarini D, Pereira A.L, de Oliveira A, Christoff Ade O, Linde G.A, do Valle J.S, Colauto N.B, Acco A. Can J Physiol Pharmacol. 2010;88(1):21-7

22. Inhibitory mechanisms of *Agaricus blazei* Murill on the growth of prostate cancer *in vitro* and *in vivo*. Yu C.H, Kan S.F, Shu C.H, Lu TJ, Sun-Hwang L, Wang P.S. J Nutr Biochem. 2009;20(10):753-64

23. Immunomodulating activity of *Agaricus brasiliensis* KA21 in mice and in human volunteers. Liu Y, Fukuwatari Y, Okumura K, Takeda K, Ishibashi KI, Furukawa M, Ohno N, Mori K, Gao M, Motoi M. Evid Based Complement Alternat Med. 2008;5(2):205-219

24. Natural killer cell activity and quality of life were improved by consumption of a mushroom extract, *Agaricus blazei* Murill Kyowa, in gynecological cancer patients undergoing chemotherapy. Ahn W.S, et al. Int J Gynecol Cancer 2004;14(4):589-594

25. Clinical observation on treatment of acute non lymphocytic leukaemia with Agaricus blazei. X. Tian, Z. Lun and H. Ito. J. Lanzhou Med. Coll. 20 (1994), pp. 169–171

26. Observation on treatment effect of *Agaricus blazei* against alimentary tract tumour. Wang J., Mou X.M. and Cheng R.Z. Gansu Med J. 1994;13:5–7

27. White button mushroom phytochemicals inhibit aromatase activity and breast cancer cell proliferation. Grube B.J, Eng E.T, Kao Y.C, Kwon A, Chen S. J Nutr. 2001;131(12):3288-93

28. Anti-aromatase activity of phytochemicals in white button mushrooms (*Agaricus bisporus*). Chen S, Oh S.R, Phung S, Hur G, Ye J.J, Kwok S.L, Shrode G.E, Belury M, Adams L.S, Williams D. Cancer Res. 2006;66(24):12026-34

29. Medicinal properties and clinical effects of culinary-medicinal mushroom *Agaricus blazei* Murrill (Agaricomycetideae) (Review). Mizuno T. Int J Med Mushr 2002;4:299–312

30. *Agaricus blazei* (Himematsutake) does not alter the development of rat diethylnitrosamine-initiated hepatic preneoplastic foci. Barbisan L.F, Spinardi-Barbisan A.L, Moreira E.L, Salvadori D.M, Ribeiro L.R, da Eira A.F, de Camargo J.L. Cancer Sci. 2003;94(2):188-92

31. Screening for *in vitro* and *in vivo* antitumour activities of the mushroom *Agaricus blazei*. Ziliotto L, Pinheiro F, Barbisan L.F, Rodrigues M.A. Nutr Cancer. 2009;61(2):245-50

32. Variation of the antimutagenicity effects of water extracts of *Agaricus blazei* Murrill *in vitro*. Guterrez Z.R, Mantovani M.S, Eira A.F, Ribeiro L.R, Jordão B.Q. Toxicol *in vitro*. 2004;18(3):301-9

33. Effects of the medicinal mushroom *Agaricus blazei* Murill on immunity, infection and cancer. Hetland G, Johnson E, Lyberg T, Bernardshaw S, Tryggestad A.M, Grinde B. Scand J Immunol. 2008;68(4):363-70

34. An extract of the medicinal mushroom *Agaricus blazei* Murill can protect against allergy. Ellertsen L.K, Hetland G. Clin Mol Allergy. 2009:5;7-6

35. The mushroom *Agaricus blazei* Murill extract normalizes liver function in patients with chronic hepatitis B. Hsu C.H, Hwang K.C, Chiang Y.H, Chou P. J Altern Complement Med. 2008;14(3):299-301

36. Clinical utility of ABCL (Agaricus Mushroom Extract) treatment for C-type hepatitis. Jpn Pharmacol Ther. 2002;30:103-7

37. Observation on the treatment effect of *Agaricus blazei* to the liver function of chronic hepatitis patients. Wang L. and Ma H. J Lanzhou Med Coll. 2004;20:24–26

38. An alternative medicine, *Agaricus blazei*, may have induced severe hepatic dysfunction in cancer patients. Mukai H, Watanabe T, Ando M, Katsumata N. Jpn J Clin Oncol. 2006 Dec;36(12):808-10

39. Cheilitis due to *Agaricus blazei* Murill mushroom extract. Suehiro M, Katoh N, Kishimoto S. Contact Dermatitis. May 2007;56(5): 293-294

Antrodia camphorata
(Antrodia cinnamomea)

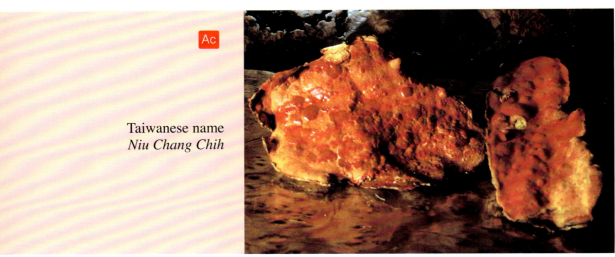

Taiwanese name
Niu Chang Chih

© 2010 Well Shine Biotechnology, Taiwan

This native Taiwanese mushroom is starting to attract interest because of the exceptionally high concentration of its triterpenoid compounds and their structural diversity. Other important bioactive compounds include polysaccharides, maleic/succinic acid derivatives, benzenoids and benzoquinone derivatives[1].

In the wild *A. camphorata* grows solely on the tree *Cinnamomum kanehirai*, a species of cinnamon that grows at altitudes of between 450 and 2,000m in the mountains of Taiwan. As the fruiting body only develops fully once the tree is dead, in the past many trees were felled to supply demand for this unique and extremely lucrative mushroom (wild *A. camphorata* fetches up to US$15,000/kg) and this, coupled with the fact that *C. kanehirai* itself is highly sought for furniture manufacture, has led to over-exploitation, with the result that *C. kanehirai* is now protected by the Taiwanese government[2].

To replace the wild-collected material, commercial cultivation of *A. camphorata* has been developed using a variety of techniques to produce either cultivated fruiting body, pure mycelium (grown by liquid fermentation), or mycelial biomass (mycelium and residual substrate). Levels of triterpenes are highest in the fruiting body products, which are also the most expensive, and lowest in the biomass products, with liquid fermentation mycelial products offering a cost-effective intermediate option.

A. camphorata has a wide range of traditional indications, including: alcohol intoxication, cancer, hypertension, fatigue, viral infection and liver disease.

HEPATOPROTECTIVE - The use of *A. camphorata* by Taiwanese natives to counter the adverse effects of excessive alcohol consumption was first reported by a traditional Chinese medicine doctor, Wu-Sha in 1773. In animal experiments both the fruiting body and mycelium have been shown to protect against alcohol-induced hepatitis and liver steatosis (fatty liver), as well as CCl4 and cytokine induced liver damage, ameliorating increases in AST, ALT and ALP levels and histopathological changes in a dose-dependent manner with no observed lesions[2,3].

A. camphorata fruiting bodies also inhibited alcohol-induced rises in cholesterol and hepatic lipids in rats with moderate effect at a dose of 0.025g/kg and increased efficacy at a dose of 0.1g/kg [4].

Separately it has been shown that *A. camphorata* possesses strong antioxidant activity and it has been suggested that this is a major contributor to its hepatoprotective properties[5,6]. Its antioxidant properties are correlated with the presence of total polyphenols, crude triterpenoids and the protein/polysaccharide ratio of the polysaccharide extract[7].

A. camphorata polysaccharides also show hepatoprotective and anti-hepatitis B activity[8,9], while a number of maleic/succinic acid derivatives showed potent inhibitory activity against hepatitis C protease through competitive inhibition[10].

In addition *A. camphorata* has been shown to suppress the invasive potential of liver cancer cells through inhibition of NF-kappaB[11] and to induce apoptosis in human hepatoma cells[12,13].

CANCER - As well as its effects on liver cancer, multiple *in vitro* and *in vivo* studies show inhibition of cancer cell growth and migration, together with increase in apoptosis, in various cancer cell lines including breast, prostate, liver, bladder and oral carcinoma[1,14-16].

ASTHMA - The immune modulating and anti-inflammatory actions of *A. camphorata* offer potential in asthma treatment with animal experiments showing that *A. camphorata* polysaccharides dose-dependently inhibited the development of airway hyperresponsiveness, airway eosinophilia and Th2 immune status[17].

SYSTEMIC LUPUS ERYTHEMATOSUS (SLE) - A mycelial extract of *A. camphorata* reduced urine protein and creatinine levels and suppressed changes in the kidney glomerular basement membrane (a histological hallmark of SLE) at a dose of 400mg/kg in a mouse model of SLE, suggesting ability to protect the kidney from autoimmune disease[18].

CARDIOVASCULAR DISEASE - *A. camphorata* has traditionally been used to treat a variety of heart conditions, including hypertension and atherosclerosis, and *A. camphorata* extracts have been reported to inhibit thickening of blood vessel walls and to promote vasodilation[19,20].

CLINICAL SUMMARY

Main Therapeutic Application - *Liver Disease*

Key Component - *Triterpenes, Polysaccharides*

Dose - *While the more expensive fruiting body contains the highest level of triterpenes and is preferred in Taiwan for cancer treatment, mycelium produced by liquid fermentation is increasingly available and has been shown to offer a cost effective alternative for treatment of liver conditions, with a recommended dose of 1-3g/day.*

Caution - *Patients on anti-coagulant medication.*

REFERENCES

1. Review of pharmacological effects of *Antrodia camphorata* and its bioactive compounds. Geethangili M, Tzeng Y.M. Evid Based Complement Alternat Med. 2009

2. Niuchangchih (*Antrodia camphorata*) and its potential in treating liver diseases. Ao Z.H, Xu Z.H, Lu Z.M, Xu H.Y, Zhang X.M, Dou W.F. J Ethnopharmacol. 2009;121(2):194-212

3. Further studies on the hepatoprotective effect of *Antrodia camphorata* in submerged culture on ethanol-induced acute liver injury in rats. Lu ZM, Tao WY, Xu HY, Ao ZH, Zhang XM, Xu ZH. Nat Prod Res. 2010 Jul 9:1-12

4. Fruiting body of Niuchangchih (*Antrodia camphorata*) protects livers against chronic alcohol consumption damage. Huang C.H, Chang Y.Y, Liu C.W, Kang W.Y, Lin Y.L, Chang H.C, Chen Y.C. J Agric Food Chem. 2010;58(6):3859-66

5. Antioxidative and hepatoprotective effects of *Antrodia camphorata* extract. Hsiao G, Shen M.Y, Lin K.H, Lan M.H, Wu L.Y, Chou D.S, Lin C.H, Su C.H, Sheu J.R. J Agric Food Chem. 2003; 51(11):3302-8

6. Protection of oxidative damage by aqueous extract from *Antrodia camphorate* mycelia in normal human erythrocytes. Hseu Y.C, et al. Life Sci.2002;71(4):469-482

7. Antioxidant properties of *Antrodia camphorata* in submerged culture. Song T.Y, Yen G.C. J Agric Food Chem. 2002;50(11):3322-7

8. Protective effects of a neutral polysaccharide isolated from the mycelium of *Antrodia cinnamomea* on Propionibacterium acnes and lipopolysaccharide induced hepatic injury in mice. Han H.F, Nakamura N, Zuo F, Hirakawa A, Yokozawa T, Hattori M. Chem Pharm Bull (Tokyo). 2006;54(4):496-500

9. *Antrodia camporata* polysaccharides exhibit anti-hepatitus B virus effects. Lee, I.H, Huang R.L, Chen C.T, Chen H.C, Hsu W.C & Lu M.K. FEMS Microbiol. Lett. 2002;209(1):63-67

10. Inhibitory effects of antrodins A-E from *Antrodia cinnamomea* and their metabolites on hepatitis C virus protease. Phuong do T, Ma C.M, Hattori M, Jin J.S. Phytother Res. 2009;23(4):582-4

11. *Antrodia cinnamomea* fruiting bodies extract suppresses the invasive potential of human liver cancer cell line PLC/PRF/5 through inhibition of nuclear factor kappaB pathway. Hsu Y.L, Kuo P.L, Cho C.Y, Ni W.C, Tzeng F, Ng L.T, Kuo Y.H, Lin C.C. Food Chem Toxicol. 2007;45(7):1249-57

12. Induction of apoptosis in human hepatoma cells by mycelia of *Antrodia camphorata* in submerged culture. Song T.Y, Hsu S.L, Yen G.C. J Ethnopharmacol. 2005;100(1-2):158-67

13. Mycelia from *Antrodia camphorata* in submerged culture induce apoptosis of human hepatoma HepG2 cells possibly through regulation of Fas pathway.Song T.Y, Hsu S.L, Yeh C.T, Yen G.C. J Agric Food Chem. 2005;53(14):5559-64

14. *Antrodia camphorata* extract induces replicative senescence in superficial TCC, and inhibits the absolute migration capability in invasive bladder carcinoma cells. Peng C.C, Chen K.C, Peng R.Y, Chyau C.C, Su C.H, Hsieh-Li H.M. J Ethnopharmacol. 2007;109(1):93-103

15. Inhibition of cyclooxygenase-2 and induction of apoptosis in estrogen-nonresponsive breast cancer cells by *Antrodia camphorata*. Hseu Y.C, et al. Food and Chemical Toxicology. 2006;45:1107-1115

16. Unique Formosan mushroom *Antrodia camphorata* differentially inhibits androgen-responsive LNCaP and independent PC-3 prostate cancer cell. Chen, Kuan-Chou et al. Nutrition and Cancer 2007; 57(1):111-121

17. Administration of polysaccharides from *Antrodia camphorata* modulates dendritic cell function and alleviates allergen-induced T helper type 2 responses in a mouse model of asthma. Liu K.J, Leu S.J, Su C.H, Chiang B.L, Chen Y.L, Lee Y.L. Immunology. 2010; 129(3):351-62

18. An extract of *Antrodia camphorata* mycelia attenuates the progression of nephritis in systemic lupus Erythematosus-prone NZB/W F1 mice. Chang J.M, Lee Y.R, Hung L.M, Liu S.Y, Kuo M.T, Wen W.C, Chen P. Evid Based Complement Alternat Med. 2008 Sep 2. Epub

19. A novel inhibitory effect of *Antrodia camphorata* extract on vascular smooth muscle cell migration and neointima formation in mice. Li Y.H, Chung H.C, Liu S.L, Chao T.H, Chen J.C. Int Heart J. 2009;50(2):207-20

20. The vasorelaxation of *Antrodia camphorata* mycelia: involvement of endothelial Ca(2+)-NO-cGMP pathway. Wang G.J, Tseng H.W, Chou C.J, Tsai T.H, Chen C.T, Lu M.K. Life Sci. 2003;73(21):2769-83

Armillaria mellea

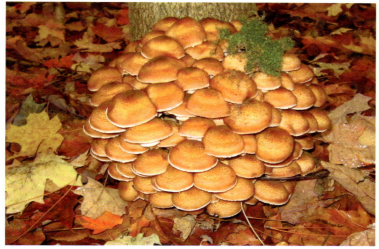

© 2010 Umberto Pascali

Chinese name
Mi Huan Jun

Japanese name
Naratake

English name
Honey Mushroom

A. mellea is a common fungus that produces edible fruiting bodies with a distinctive golden colour. A single example can grow to cover a vast area and it is reported that the largest living organism in the world is a related species of honey fungus covering an area of 2200 acres in Oregon, USA[1].

Although responsible for the death of many trees and garden shrubs, *A. mellea* is essential for the growth of other plants, including the important Chinese herb *Gastrodia elata* (*Tian Ma*), which is used to treat conditions including vertigo, dizziness, headache, stroke and convulsions and whose medical properties *A. mellea* mirrors. Indeed *A. mellea* is considered the more potent of the two with an effective dosage half that of *Tian Ma*[2].

Early reports indicated that *A. mellea* and *G. elata* shared the same active components but it is now known that they differ in their active metabolites[3].

As well as being essential for the growth of *G. elata*, it has been shown that *Armillaria* species are involved in sclerotium formation in *Polyporus umbelatus* (see *P. umbellatus* section).

A. mellea mycelium contains high levels of polysaccharides with anti-aging, immune modulating and anti-vertigo activity[4]. In addition, nucleoside analogues play a role in some of *A. mellea's* functions[5].

Several antibiotics, primarily sesquiterpene aryl esters, have been isolated from *A. mellea* and show strong action against gram-positive bacteria (*Staphylococcus, Streptococcus, Enterococcus* etc.), as well as yeasts and other fungi[6,7,8].

NEUROLOGICAL - Tablets composed of *A. mellea* mycelium are prescribed in China for treating a variety of neurological conditions including Meniere's Syndrome, vertigo, epilepsy, neurasthenia and hypertension[2,9-11].

A. mellea fermentation extract showed anti-convulsant properties, raising the seizure threshold in PTZ-induced seizures in mice[12], while an adenosine derivative from the mycelium abolished neurogenic twitch responses induced by electrical field stimulation with both pre- and post-synapse depression, as well as being found to be 1,000 times stronger than adenosine in its cerebral protecting activity[8]. In addition *A. mellea* polysaccharide extract was shown to benefit vertigo induced by machinery rotation[13].

CLINICAL SUMMARY

Main Therapeutic Application - *Meniere's Syndrome, Vertigo, Epilepsy*

Key Components - *Polysaccharides, nucleoside derivatives and sesquiterpene aryl esters*

Dose - *Mycelial tablets are used in China 3-4g/day*

REFERENCES

1. Medicinal mushrooms - an exploration of tradition, healing and culture. Hobbs C. 1986. Pub Botanica Press, Williams
2. Modernizing chinese medicine - the case of *armillaria* as gastrodia substitute. Dharmananda S. www.itmonline.org/arts/gastrodia.htm
3. Tian ma, an ancient Chinese herb, offers new options for the treatment of epilepsy and other conditions. Ojemann L.M, Nelson W.L, Shin D.S, Rowe A.O, Buchanan R.A. Epilepsy & Behavior. 2006;8(2):376-383
4. The cultivation, bioactive components and pharmacological effects of *Armillaria mellea*. Gao L.W, Li W.Y, Zhao Y.L and Wang J.W. Afr J Biotech. 2009;8(25):7383-7390
5. A novel N6-substituted adenosine isolated from mi huan jun (*Armillaria mellea*) as a cerebral-protecting compound. Watanabe N, Obuchi T, Tamai M, Araki H, Omura S, Yang JS, Yu D.Q, Liang X.T, Huan J.H. Planta Med. 1990;56(1):48-52
6. Armillaric acid, a new antibiotic produced by *Armillaria mellea*. Obuchi T, Kondoh H, Watanabe N, Tamai M, Omura S, Yang J.S, Liang X.T. Planta Med. 1990;56(2):198-201
7. Antimicrobial and antioxidant activities of mycelia of 10 wild mushroom species. Kalyoncu F, Oskay M, Sağlam H, Erdoğan TF, Tamer A.U. J Med Food. 2010;13(2):415-94
8. Antibacterial sesquiterpene aryl esters from *Armillaria mellea*. Donnelly D.M, Abe F, Coveney D, Fukuda N, O'Reilly J, Polonsky J, Prange T. J Nat Prod. 1985;48(1):10-6
9. To use *Armillaria* fungus tablet to replace gastrodia tuber in treating 45 cases with syndrome of deficiency of yin and flourishing yang, Chinese Journal of Medicine, 1977;8:473-474
10. Observation on curative effects of *Armillaria mellea* fungus tablet in treating 100 cases of neurasthenia and hypertension, etc. Zhou Linshen. Journal of New Medicine, 1978;10:13
11. Curative effects of gastrodia tuber *Armellaria* fungus tablet in treating some diseases of the nervous system. Jiangsu Journal of TCM. 1980;1:35-37
12. Pharmacological actions of gastrodia watery preparation and fermentation liquid of *Armellaria mellea* on nervous system. Chinese Journal of Medicine. 1977;8:470-472
13. Study on the anti-vertigo function of polysaccharides of *Gastrodia elata* and polysaccharides of *Armillaria mellea*. Yu L. Shen Y.S, Miao H.C. Chin J Information, TCM. 2006;13:29-36

Auricularia auricula
(Auricularia polytricha)

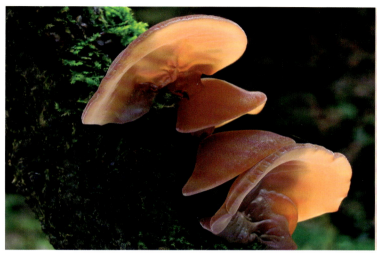

Japanese Name
Kikurage

Chinese Name
Mu Er / Wood Ear

English Name
Jews Ear / Judas' Ear

© 2010 Jaroslav Malý

A. auricula grows throughout Europe, Asia and the United States and is highly valued in Asian cooking for its crunchy, rubbery texture. A type of jelly fungus, it produces fruiting bodies that are translucent, brown in colour and 'ear' shaped, hence its Chinese name 'Wood Ear'. Both *A. auricula* and *A. polytricha* are considered as species of *Mu Er* in Chinese medicine and today are used interchangeably[1].

In common with other jelly fungi, *A. auricula* fruiting bodies contain high levels of polysaccharides and these are the main bioactive component, although phenols have been shown to contribute to the total antioxidant capacity[2].

A. auricula is of particular interest as a functional food for the elderly, with polysaccharide extracts showing particular promise and having been developed as functional food additives for bread[3].

ANTI-INFLAMMATORY - *A. auricula* polysaccharides have anti-inflammatory activity, which correlates with *A. auricula*'s traditional use for soothing irritated or inflamed mucous membranes[4].

ANTIOXIDANT - *A. auricula* extracts show strong antioxidant properties with a positive correlation between levels of phenols and antioxidant capacity[5-7].

ANTI-THROMBOTIC - Polysaccharide extracts of *A. auricula* inhibit platelet aggregation and increase clotting times *in vitro* and *in vivo*. Its anti-coagulant activity was due to catalysis of thrombin inhibition by antithrombin but not by heparin cofactor II[8,9].

ANTI-CHOLESTEROL - *A. auricula* polysaccharides have been shown to lower blood total cholesterol (TC), triglyceride and LDL levels and enhance the level of blood HDL, as well as HDL/TC and HDL/LDL ratios at 5% of feed in rats suffering from hyperlipidemia[10-12].

CARDIOPROTECTIVE - Together with *A. auricula*'s general antioxidant properties, *A. auricula* polysaccharides show strong cardio-protective action, especially in aged mice, enhancing the activity of superoxide dismutase and reducing lipid peroxidation[13,14].

CLINICAL SUMMARY

Main Therapeutic application - *Cardiovascular support*

Key Component - *Polysaccharides*

Dose - *2-3g/day polysaccharide extract*

Caution - *Patients on anti-coagulant medication. Owing to possible anti-fertility effects it is recommended that A. auricula not be taken by pregnant or lactating women or those planning to conceive[15].*

REFERENCES

1. Hobbs C. Medicinal Mushrooms - An Exploration of Tradition, Healing and Culture. 1986. Botanica Press, Williams, Oregon

2. Research progress in *Auricularia auricula* polysaccharide. Huang X.G, Quan Y.L, Guan B, Hu Y. Science and Technology of Cereals, Oils and Foods. 2010-01

3. Evaluation of antioxidant property and quality of breads containing *Auricularia auricula* polysaccharide flour. Fan L, Zhang S, Yu L. Li Ma Food Chemistry, 2007

4. Polysaccharides in fungi. XIV. Anti-inflammatory effect of the polysaccharides from the fruit bodies of several fungi. Ukai S, Kiho T, Hara C, Kuruma I, Tanaka Y. J Pharmacobiodyn. 1983;6(12):983-90

5. Antioxidant capacity of fresh and processed fruit bodies and mycelium of *Auricularia auricula-judae* (Fr.) Quél. Kho Y.S, Vikineswary S, Abdullah N, Kuppusamy U.R, Oh H.I. J Med Food. 2009;12(1):167-74

6. Antioxidant and nitric oxide synthase activation properties of *Auricularia auricula*. Acharya K, Samui K, Rai M, Dutta B.B, Acharya R. Indian J Exp Biol. 2004;42(5):538-40

7. Antioxidant activity of submerged cultured mycelium extracts of higher *Basidiomycetes* mushrooms, Asatiani M et al. Int J Med Mush. 2007;9

8. The nontoxic mushroom *Auricularia auricula* contains a polysaccharide with anticoagulant activity mediated by antithrombin. Yoon S.J, Yu M.A, Pyun Y.R, Hwang J.K, Chu D.C, Juneja L.R, Mourão P.A. Thromb Res. 2003;112(3):151-18

9. Inhibition of human and rat platelet aggregation by extracts of Mu-er (*Auricularia auricula*). Thromb Haemost. Agarwal K.C, Russo F.X, Parks R.E Jr. 1982;48(2):162-5

10. Effect of polysaccharide from *Auricularia auricula* on blood lipid metabolism and lipoprotein lipase activity of ICR mice fed a cholesterol-enriched diet. Chen G, Luo YC, Li BP, Li B, Guo Y, Li Y, Su W, Xiao ZL. J Food Sci. 2008 Aug;73(6):H103-8

11. The hypocholesterolemic effect of two edible mushrooms: *Auricularia auricula* (tree-ear) and Tremella fuciformis (white jelly-leaf) in hypercholesterolemic rats. Kaneda T and Tokuda S. Nutrition Research. 1996;1699(10):1721-1725

12. Isolation and purification of polysaccharides from wood ear (*Auricularia auricular*) and their hypoglycemic, hypolipidemic and antioxidant activities. Yi M.A, Tang J, Han C. 2005 IFT Annual Meeting. ift.confex.com 18B-13

13. Chemical characterization of *Auricularia auricula* polysaccharides and its pharmacological effect on heart antioxidant enzyme activities and left ventricular function in aged mice. Wu Q, Tan Z, Liu H, Gao L, Wu S, Luo J, Zhang W, Zhao T, Yu J, Xu X. Int J Biol Macromol. 2010 Apr 1;46(3):284-8

14. *Auricularia auricular* polysaccharide protects myocardium against ischemia/reperfusion injury. Ye TM, Qian LB, Cui J, Wang HP, Ye ZG, Xia Q. Zhongguo Ying Yong Sheng Li Xue Za Zhi. 2010 May;26(2):154-8

15. Anti-fertility action of *Auricularia auricula* polysaccharide. He B. Chen Q. Zhongguo Yaoke Daxue Xuebao. 1991;22:48-49

Cordyceps sinensis

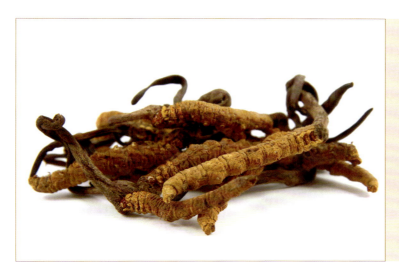

Cs

Japanese name
Tochukas

Chinese name
Dong Chong Xia Cao

English name
Caterpillar Fungus

Cordyceps is unique among the medicinal mushrooms in growing on an insect host rather than a plant host. To date over 700 species of cordyceps have been identified worldwide, in most cases growing parasitically on their insect hosts. However, it appears likely that in some cases a symbiotic relationship exists whereby the insect host derives a selective advantage from the fungal anamorph (the fungus growing in a single cell form), especially in marginal environments where energy efficiency is at a premium, such as the high Tibetan plateau above 3,000m where the main species used traditionally, *Cordyceps sinensis*, occurs naturally[1].

Although traditionally harvested cordyceps is still available, the vast majority of cordyceps on the market today is cultivated on non-insect, grain-based substrates leading to improved quality control and affordability. Despite the commercially cultivated cordyceps being grown on a different substrate from the wild collected cordyceps, HPLC analysis shows identical chemical profiles and the two are seen to be interchangeable clinically[2].

As well as polysaccharides and lipids, *Cordyceps species* contain a large number of nucleoside analogues, prominent among which is cordycepin, 3-deoxyadenosine, which differs from adenosine in the absence of oxygen at the 3 position of its ribose part[3]. Because of its close similarity to adenosine some enzymes cannot distinguish between the two and it is able to participate in certain biochemical reactions, including RNA/DNA synthesis, where its incorporation leads to the termination of the RNA/DNA molecule, there being no oxygen to bond with the next nucleotide[4-7].

This ability to interrupt RNA/DNA synthesis has led to the use of such nucleoside analogues, termed reverse transcriptase inhibitors, in the treatment of viral infections, including HIV and Hepatitis, as well as cancer, under pharmaceutical names including AZT (Retrovir), Videx and Epivir. In normal healthy cells such reverse transcriptase inhibitors are out-competed by the corresponding nucleoside but in rapidly dividing cancer cells and virally infected cells they are able to exert effective inhibition of replication.

Adenosine in the form of adenosine monophosphate and adenosine triphosphate also plays a central role in energy metabolism and cyclic nucleotides including cAMP play an important role in signal transduction and regulation of hormone production, actions which correlate well with the observed activity of cordyceps in these areas.

ANTI-AGING - *C. sinensis* has traditionally been used as a supplement for the elderly and those recovering from long illness. Studies with the Cordyceps Cs-4 strain in healthy elderly subjects showed significant increases in oxygen uptake, aerobic capacity and resistance to fatigue.

Experimental evidence based on polysaccharide extracts indicates that *C. sinensis* is also able to improve brain function and antioxidative enzyme activity (superoxide dismutase, glutathione peroxidase and catalase), which, together with its beneficial effect on cardiovascular function, makes it an excellent supplement for the elderly[8].

ATHLETIC PERFORMANCE - The use of *C. sinensis*, together with other supplements, by the record breaking Chinese athletes of the early 1990s has attracted considerable interest in its potential to enhance athletic performance.

A 1996 study on long distance runners reported a significant improvement in 71% of participants and both *C. sinensis* and a closely related species, *C. militaris*, have been shown to increase endurance in animal models. Studies on sedentary humans also show a significant increase in energy output and oxygen capacity[9-12].

However, three subsequent human studies have failed to demonstrate any effect on performance in competitive cyclists or other professional athletes and it has been suggested that this may be because such athletes are already operating at or close to their maximum aerobic capacity[13,14].

SEXUAL FUNCTION - *C. sinensis* produces clear benefits for male sexual hypofunction when taken over a period of time. Anecdotal evidence and reports from China also indicate possible benefits for female libido.

Based on animal studies *C. sinensis* and related species have a clear effect on increasing levels of male sex hormones, improving testes morphology, sperm quantity and quality. *In vitro* research indicates that cordyceps affects the signal transduction pathway of steroidogenesis after the formation of cAMP[15-19].

FERTILITY - *C. sinensis* is increasingly being used by leading specialists in the field of infertility and clinical evidence suggests that cordyceps has a beneficial impact on female fertility and the success of IVF. In part this may be due to its ability to stimulate 17β-estradiol (oestrogen) production, through increased StAR (steroidogenic acute regulatory protein) and aromatase expression[20]. In common with other mushrooms, cordyceps' ability to regulate immune function and in particular NK cell activity may also play a part.

The ability of *C. sinensis* to increase oestrogen production also has potential for the management of postmenopausal osteoporosis[21].

DIABETES - Experimental evidence indicates that *C. sinensis* is able to:
- Trigger release of insulin
- Increase hepatic glucokinase
- Increase sensitivity of cells to insulin

In one randomized trial 95% of patients treated with 3g/day *C. sinensis* biomass saw improvements in their blood sugar profile compared with 54% treated by other methods. In addition it has been reported that consumption of 4.5g/day *C. sinensis* biomass by patients with alcohol induced diabetes also produced a reduced desire for alcohol[2,22-25].

Recent evidence indicates that cordycepin and related nucleoside derivatives play an active role in the anti-diabetic action of *C. sinensis*[26].

HEPATOPROTECTIVE - Animal studies have shown the ability of *C. sinensis* to inhibit hepatic fibrosis and help restore liver function. One clinical study using 3g/day *C. sinensis* biomass to treat alcohol-induced liver steatosis in 14 patients showed reductions of 70% in AST levels, 63% in ALT levels and 64% in GGT levels over a 90 day period[27,28].

KIDNEY PROTECTIVE - *C. sinensis* has traditionally been considered to possess the ability to support the kidneys and 3.5g/day has been shown to both improve kidney function in patients with chronic renal failure and speed recovery in patients with gentamycin induced kidney damage[2].

RESPIRATORY DISEASE - *C. sinensis* has traditionally been used to treat respiratory ailments and is reported to be beneficial for asthma and COPD[2].

ANTI-VIRAL - As mentioned above, the nucleoside analogues present in *Cordyceps species* are able to inhibit viral replication. At the same time the polysaccharides in cordyceps modulate the immune response to viral infections. This combination of enhanced immune response and interrupted viral replication makes cordyceps one of the most effective mushrooms for tackling chronic viral infections[5,6].

ANTI-CANCER - *C. sinensis* also shows promise for cancer treatment and a growing body of *in vitro* evidence supports the ability of the nucleoside derivatives, particularly cordycepin, to induce apoptosis, inhibit nuclear factor kappaB (NF-kB) and activator protein-1 (AP-1) production and increase levels of Th1 promoting cytokines[29-33].

CLINICAL SUMMARY

Main Therapeutic Applications - *Fertility and sexual function, Energy, Diabetes, Lung Function, Kidney Support, Liver Disorders*

Key Component - *Nucleoside derivatives*

Dose - *Cordyceps' unique properties are principally those of its nucleoside derivatives and as these are largely excreted (research on C. militaris shows that 98% of cordycepin is secreted into the growth medium[34]) biomass products offer the natural dosage format for cordyceps. 3-6g/day biomass is used in most cases while doses of up to 50g/day cordyceps biomass have been reported to give good results in a range of cancers[2].*

The finding that other species of cordyceps produce higher levels of nucleoside derivatives than C. sinensis has also led to the development of hybrid strains and the use of growing conditions that replicate those in the natural environment in order to maximise their production[35,36].

Caution - *Hormone dependent cancers (prostate and breast) due to increased levels of oestrogen and testosterone.*

REFERENCES

1. *Cordyceps* fungi: natural products, pharmacological functions and developmental products. Zhou X, Gong Z, Su Y, Lin J, Tang K. J Pharm Pharmacol. 2009;61(3):279-91

2. Medicinal value of the caterpillar fungi species of the genus *Cordyceps* (Fr.) Link (Ascomycetes). A Review. Holliday J, Cleaver M. Int J Med Mushr, 2008;10(3):219–234

3. Analysis of the main nucleosides in *Cordyceps sinensis* by LC/ESI-MS. Xie J.W, Huang L.F, Hu W, He Y.B, Wong K.P. Molecules. 2010;15(1):305-14

4. Some biologically active substances from a mycelial biomass of medicinal 'Caterpillar fungus' *Cordyceps sinensis* (Berk.) Sacc. (Ascomycetes). Smirnov D.A, Babitskaya V.G, Puchkova T.A, Shcherba V.V, Bisko N.A, Poyedinok N.L. Int J Med Mushr. 2009;11(1):80

5. Effect of Cordycepin Triphosphate on in vitro RNA synthesis by plant viral replicases. White J.L, Dawson W.O. J Virol. 1979;29(2):811-814

6. Cordycepin interferes with 3' end formation in yeast independently of its potential to terminate RNA chain elongation. RNA. 2009;15(5):837-49

7. Cordycepin inhibits (collagen induced) human platelet platelet aggregation in a cAMP- and cGMP-dependent manner. Eur J Pharmacol. 2007;558:43-51

8. Antiaging effect of *Cordyceps sinensis* extract. Ji D.B, Ye J, Li C.L, Wang Y.H, Zhao J, Cai S.Q. Phytother Res. 2009;23(1):116-22

9. Increased aerobic capacity in healthy elderly humans given a fermentation product of *Cordyceps* CS-4. Xiao, Y.; Huang, X. Z.; Chen, G.; Wang, M. B.; Zhu, J. S.; Cooper, C. B. FACSM Medicine & Science in Sports & Exercise: May 1999; 31(5):174

10. Randomized double-blind placebo-controlled clinical trial and assessment of fermentation product of *Cordyceps sinensis* (Cs-4) in enhancing aerobic capacity and respiratory function of the healthy elderly volunteers. Xiao Y, Huang X.Z and Zhu J.S. Chinese Journal of Integrative Medicine. 2004;10,3:187-192

11. Effect of medicinal plant extracts on forced swimming capacity in mice. Jung K, Kim IH, Han D. J Ethnopharmacol. 2004 Jul;93(1):75-81

12. CordyMax enhances aerobic capability, endurance performance, and exercise metabolism in healthy, mid-age to elderly sedentary humans. JS Zhu, JM Rippe - Gerontology, 2001

13. *Cordyceps Sinensis* Supplementation Does Not Improve Endurance Performance in Competitive Cyclists. Parcell A.C, Smith J.M, Schulthies S.S, Myrer J.W, Fellingham G. Medicine & Science in Sports & Exercise: 2002;34(5):231
14. Does *Cordyceps sinensis* Ingestion Aid Athletic Performance? TB Walker. Strength and Conditioning Journal, 2006
15. Effect of *Cordyceps militaris* supplementation on sperm production, sperm motility and hormones in Sprague-Dawley rats. Am J Chin Med. 2008;36(5):849-59
16. *in vivo* and *in vitro* stimulatory effects of *Cordyceps sinensis* on testosterone production in mouse Leydig cells. Life Sci. 2003 Sep 5;73(16):2127-36
17. Influence of *Cordyceps Sinensis* on Reproduction and Testis Morphology in Mice. Shenzhen Journal of Integrated Chinese and Western Medicine. 2005-6
18. Improvement of sperm production in subfertile boars by *Cordyceps militaris* supplement. Am J Chin Med. 2007;35(4):631-41
19. Estrogenic Substances from the Mycelia of Medicinal Fungus *Cordyceps ophioglossoides* (Ehrh.) Fr. (Ascomycetes). Hirokazu Kawagishi, Kentaro Okamura, Fumio Kobayashi, Noriko Kinjo. IntJMedMushr.v6.i3.40 2004
20. Upregulation of Steroidogenic Enzymes and Ovarian 17β-Estradiol in Human Granulosa-Lutein Cells by Cordyceps sinensis Mycelium. Biology of Reproduction May 1, 2004 vol. 70 no. 5 1358-1364
21. The Co-effect of *Cordyceps sinensis* and Strontium on Osteoporosis in Ovariectomized Osteopenic Rats. Qi W, Yan YB, Wang PJ, Lei W. Biol Trace Elem Res. 2010 May 5
22. Hypoglycemic Activity of a Polysaccharide (CS-F30) from the Cultural Mycelium of *Cordyceps sinensis* and Its Effect on Glucose Metabolism in Mouse Liver. Kiho T, et al. Biol Pharm Bull. Feb1996;19(2):294-96
23. Structural Features and Hypoglycemic Activity of a Polysaccharide (CS-F10) from the Cultured Mycelium of *Cordyceps sinensis*. Kiho T, Ookubo K, Usui S, et al. Biol Pharm Bull. Sep1999;22(9):966-70
24. Anti-hyperglycemic activity of natural and fermented in rats with diabetes induced by nicotinamide and streptozotocin. Lo HC, Hsu TH, Tu ST, Lin KC. Am J Chin Med. 2006;34(5):819-32
25. Hypoglycemic activity of polysaccharide, with antioxidation, isolated from cultured *Cordyceps* mycelia. Li SP, Zhang GH, Zeng Q, Huang ZG, Wang YT, Dong TT, Tsim KW. Phytomedicine. 2006 Jun;13(6):428-33
26. Cordycepin Suppresses Expression of Diabetes Regulating Genes by Inhibition of Lipopolysaccharide-induced Inflammation in Macrophages. Shin S, Lee S, Kwon J, Moon S, Lee S, Lee CK, Cho K, Ha NJ, Kim K. Immune Netw. 2009 Jun;9(3):98-105
27. Inhibitive Effect of *Cordyceps sinensis* on Experimental Hepatic Fibrosis and its Possible Mechanism- Liu YK, Shen W. Department of Gastrointerology, the Second Affiliated Hosptial, Chongqing University of Medicial Sciences, Chongqing 400010, Chinga World J Gastroenterol. 2003. 2003 Mar;9(3):529-33
28. Dynamical Influence of *Cordyceps sinensis* on the Activity of Hepatic Insulinase of Experiemental Liver Cirrhosis-Zhang X, Liu YK, Shen W, Shen DM. Hepatobiliary Pancreat Dis Int. 2004 Beb;3(1):99-101
29. RNA-directed agent, cordycepin, induces cell death in multiple myeloma cells. Chen LS, Stellrecht CM, Gandhi V. Br J Haematol. 2008 Mar;140(6):682-391. 30. Antitumour activity of Cordycepin in mice. Clin Exp Pharmacol Physiol. 31, S51-S53. 2004
30. Cordycepin inhibits protein synthesis and cell adhesion through effects on signal transduction. J Biol Chem. 2010 Jan 22;285(4):2610-21
31. Effect of cordycepin on interleukin-10 production of human peripheral blood mononuclear cells. European Journal of Pharmacology, volume 453, Issues 2-3, 25 October 2002, Pages 309-317
32. Cordycepin suppresses TNF-alpha-induced invasion, migration and matrix metalloproteinase-9 expression in human bladder cancer cells. Lee EJ, Kim WJ, Moon SK. Phytother Res. 2010 Jun 17
33. Role of Cordycepin and Adenosine on the Phenotypic Switch of Macrophages via Induced Anti-inflammatory Cytokines. Shin S, Moon S, Park Y, Kwon J, Lee S, Lee CK, Cho K, Ha NJ, Kim K.Immune Netw. 2009 Dec;9(6):255-64
34. Production of cordycepin by surface culture using the medicinal mushroom *Cordyceps militaris*. Masuda M, Urabe E, Akihiko Sakurai A, Sakakibara M. Enzyme and Microbial Technology 2006;39(4):641-646
35. Analysis of Quality and Techniques for Hybridization of Medicinal Fungus *Cordyceps sinensis* (Berk.)Sacc. (Ascomycetes). Holliday JC, Megan LP, Dinesh P. Int J Med Mushr. 2004;6(2)
36. Determination of nucleosides and nucleobases in different species of *Cordyceps* by capillary electrophoresis-mass spectrometry. Yang FQ, Ge L, Yong JW, Tan SN, Li SP. J Pharm Biomed Anal. 2009 Oct 15;50(3):307-14

Flammulina velutipes

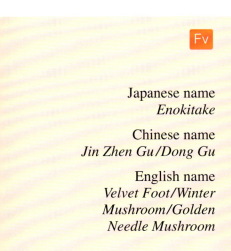

Japanese name
Enokitake

Chinese name
Jin Zhen Gu/Dong Gu

English name
Velvet Foot/Winter Mushroom/Golden Needle Mushroom

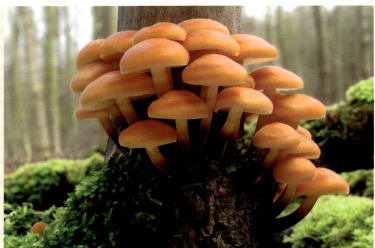

© 2010 Jaroslav Malý

A common culinary mushroom, *F. velutipes* was the second earliest mushroom to be cultivated (cultivation started around 800 AD, after *Auricularia auricula* ~600 AD, and before *Lentinus edodes* ~1000 AD).

It shows considerable clinical promise, especially for cancer prevention protocols.

A study of 174,505 inhabitants of the Nagano area of Japan compared the cancer death rates among *F. velutipes* farmers with rates in the general population over a 15 year period (1972-86) and found that the *F. velutipes* farmers had a much lower death rate of 97.1 per 100,000, compared to 160.1 per 100,000 in the general population, with the suggestion that this was due to increased consumption of *F. velutipes*[1].

Following on from the above a case-control study investigated the relationship between risk reduction of stomach cancer and intake of edible mushrooms in the same prefecture from 1998 to 2002. While the odds ratio (OR) of subjects who were eating hardly any mushrooms or mushrooms less than once a week was 1.00, consumption of *F. velutipes* more than three times a week produced a reduction to 0.66 (the OR of those taking *Lentinus edodes* (Shiitake) more than three times a week was 0.95)[2].

As well as immunomodulatory polysaccharides[3,4], *F. velutipes* is notable for its high protein content (31.2%) and large number of protein rich components with strong immuno-modulatory and anti-cancer activity[5-9].

F. velutipes extracts also demonstrate strong tyrosinase inhibition[10].

CANCER - *F. velutipes* extracts show exceptionally high anti-cancer activity *in vitro*. In one study of extracts from 38 mushrooms carried out by Bastyr University, *F. velutipes* had one of the highest levels of inhibitory activity against two oestrogen-dependent and one oestrogen independent breast cancer cell lines[11]. In a separate study of aqueous extracts from 20 mushrooms and 3 mushroom polysaccharides, the aqueous extract from *F. velutipes*, together with that from *Pleurotus ostreatus*, showed the highest level of cytotoxic activity against androgen-independent prostate cancer cells[12].

In vivo, EA6, a protein-bound polysaccharide isolated from the fruiting body of *F. velutipes*, augmented humoral immunity, cellular immunity, and IL-2 production in mice bearing Meth-A fibrosarcoma at 10mg/kg and administration after surgery remarkably inhibited growth of the rechallenged Meth-A solid tumour, while Proflammin (90% protein, 10% polysaccharide) isolated from the mycelium of *F. velutipes*, abolished suppression of immunocompetence after cryosurgery at 10mg/kg/day[13].

Another protein from *F. velutipes*, Fve, protected mice against liver cancer through activation of both innate and adaptive immune responses when administered orally at a dose of 10mg/kg[14].

In clinical studies EEM, a combination of extracts from *F. velutipes* and *Hypsizygus marmoreus*, revealed superior results to MPA (methyl-acetoxy-progesterone) on the cachexia of advanced cancer patients with better clinical response, performance status (PS), and quality of life (QOL). EEM supplementation in combination with anti-cancer drugs improved the clinical response rate, PS, and QOL of advanced cancer patients compared to patients treated with anticancer drugs alone. EEM supplementation also reduced precancerous lesions on the oesophageal mucosa[2].

ANTI-VIRAL - Co-administration of Fve, a protein from *F. velutipes*, with immunization against HPV-16 led to 60% of mice remaining tumour-free 167 days after challenge with tumour cells compared to 20% of those receiving immunization alone. The co-immunized mice showed enhanced production of HPV-16 E7 oncoprotein-specific antibodies as well as expansion of HPV-16 E7-specific interferon (IFN)-gamma-producing CD4(+) and CD8(+) T cells compared to mice immunized with HPV-16 E7 alone[15].

Proteins from *F. velutipes* also show direct anti-viral activity, including ribosome inactivating activity and inhibition of HIV-1 reverse transcriptase, beta-glucosidase and beta-glucuronidase[16].

FOOD ALLERGIES - Mice orally given five daily 200 μg doses of protein from *F. velutipes* before and after each of two intraperitoneal injections of ovalbumin significantly reduced symptoms of anaphylaxis and levels of plasma histamine on subsequent oral challenge with ovalbumin and demonstrated an impaired OVA-specific IgE response with a Th1-predominant cytokine profile[17]. Other research has demonstrated the ability of the *F. velutipes* protein Fve to enhance eosinophil apoptosis, with therapeutic implications for eosinophil-related allergic inflammation, and of an ethanol extract to suppress hypersensitive immune response[18-20].

CLINICAL SUMMARY

Main Therapeutic Application - *Dietary supplementation in patients at risk of cancer or with chrome viral conditions*

Key Component - *Proteins and polysaccharides*

Dose - *F. velutipes fruiting body contains high levels of the therapeutically active proteins at a reasonable cost and is the preferred dosage form in most cases. 3-5g dried fruiting body equates to 30-50g fresh mushroom.*

REFERENCES

1. Beneficial effects of edible and medicinal mushrooms on health care. Ikekawa T - Int J Med Mushr. 2001;3(4):8-12
2. Cancer Risk Reduction by Intake of Mushrooms and Clinical Studies on EEM. Ikekawa T. Int J Med Mush. 2005;7(3):347
3. Inhibitory activity of polysaccharide extracts from three kinds of edible fungi on proliferation of human hepatoma SMMC-7721 cell and mouse implanted S180 tumour. Jiang S.M, Xiao Z.M, Xu Z.H. World J Gastroenterol. 1999;5(5):404-407
4. Investigation of immunomodulating activity of the medicinal mushroom *Flammulina velutipes* (Curt.: Fr.) P. Karst. *in vitro*. Cytokine induction by fruiting body extract Badalyan S, Hambardzumyan L.A. Int J Med Mush. 2001;3(2-3):110-111
5. Effect of *Flammulina velutipes* polysaccharides on production of cytokines by murine immunocytes and serum levels of cytokines in tumour-bearing mice. Chang H.L, Lei L.S, Yu C.L, Zhu Z.G, Chen N.N, Wu S.G. Zhong Yao Cai. 2009;32(4):561-3
6. FIP-fve stimulates interferon-gamma production via modulation of calcium release and PKC-alpha activation. Ou C.C, Hsiao Y.M, Wu W.J, Tasy G.J, Ko J.L, Lin M.Y. J Agric Food Chem. 2009;57(22):11008-13
7. Fungal immunomodulatory protein from *Flammulina velutipes* induces interferon-gamma production through p38 mitogen-activated protein kinase signaling pathway. Wang P.H, Hsu C.I, Tang S.C, Huang Y.L, Lin J.Y, Ko J.L. J Agric Food Chem. 2004;52(9):2721-5
8. Flammulin: a novel ribosome-inactivating protein from fruiting bodies of the winter mushroom *Flammulina velutipes*. Wang H.X, Ng T.B. Biochem Cell Biol. 2000;78(6):699-702
9. High processing tolerances of immunomodulatory proteins in Enoki and Reishi mushrooms. Tong M.H, Chien P.J, Chang H.H, Tsai M.J, Sheu F. J Agric Food Chem. 2008;56(9):3160-6
10. Isolation of 1',3'-dilinolenoyl'-2'-linoleoylglycerol with tyrosinase inhibitory activity from *Flammulina velutipes*. Jang S.G, Jeon K.S, Lee E.H, Kong W.S, Cho J.Y. J Microbiol Biotechnol. 2009;19(7):681-4
11. *in vitro* effects on proliferation, apoptosis and colony inhibition in E-dependent and ER-independent human breast cancer cells by selected mushroom species. Gu Y.H, Leonard J. Oncology Reports. 2006;15:417-423
12. Cytotoxic effect of oyster mushroom *Pleurotus ostreatus* on human Androgen-independent prostate cancer PC-3 Cells. Gu Y.H, Sivam G. J Med Food. 2006;9(2):196-204
13. Immunomodulation and antitumour activity of a mushroom product, Proflamin, isolated from *Flammulina velutipes* (W. Curt.: Fr.) Singer (Agaricomycetideae). Maruyama H, Ikekawa T. Int J Med Mushr. 2007;9(2):20
14. Oral administration of an Enoki mushroom protein FVE activates innate and adaptive immunity and induces anti-tumour activity against murine hepatocellular carcinoma. Chang H.H, Hsieh K.Y, Yeh C.H, Tu Y.P, Sheu F. Int Immunopharmacol. 2010;10(2):239-46
15. Coadministration of the fungal immunomodulatory protein FIP-Fve and a tumour-associated antigen enhanced antitumour immunity. Ding Y, Seow S.V, Huang C.H, Liew L.M, Lim Y.C, Kuo I.C, Chua K.Y. Immunology. 2009;128(1Sup):881-94
16. Isolation and characterization of velutin, a novel low-molecular-weight ribosome-inactivating protein from winter mushroom (*Flammulina velutipes*) fruiting bodies. Wang H, Ng T.B. Life Sci. 2001;68(18):2151-8
17. Oral administration of an edible-mushroom-derived protein inhibits the development of food-allergic reactions in mice. Hsieh K.Y, Hsu C, Lin J.Y, Tsai C.C, Lin R.H. Clin Exp Allergy. 2003;33(11):1595-602
18. The modulatory effect of FIP-fve on eosinophil apoptosis *in vitro* indicates that it may have some therapeutic effect on eosinophil-related allergic inflammation *in vivo*. J Formos Med Assoc. 2007;106(1):36-43
19. Eosinophil apoptosis induced by fungal immunomodulatory peptide-fve via reducing IL-5alpha receptor. Hsieh C.W, Lan J.L, Meng Q, Cheng Y.W, Huang H.M, Tsai J.J. J Formos Med Assoc. 2007;106(1):36-43
20. Inhibitory effects of edible higher Basidiomycetes mushroom extracts on mouse type IV allergy. Sano M, Yoshino K, Matsuzawa T, Ikekawa T. Int J Med Mushr. 2002;4(1):37-41

Ganoderma Lucidum

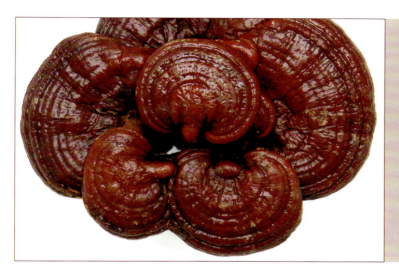

GI

Japanese name
Reishi or Mannetake (10,000 year mushroom/mushroom of immortality)

Chinese name
Ling Zhi (spirit mushroom - mushroom of spritual potency)

The most famous of all the medicinal mushrooms with annual sales of over US$2billion, *G. lucidum*'s wide-ranging health benefits are due to its combination of high polysaccharide content (Stamets reports the fruiting body to contain 41% beta-glucan) and triterpenoid compounds[1-4]. Over 130 of these have been identified, belonging to two families; ganoderic and lucidenic acids with functions including:

- Inhibiting Histamine Release
- Hepatoprotective
- Anti-hypertensive (ACE inhibiting)
- Inhibiting cholesterol synthesis
- Anti-inflammatory
- Inducing apoptosis
- Inhibiting viral induction
- Antioxidant
- Anti-tumour
- CNS sedation
- Anti-microbial
- Immune modulation

There has recently been interest in the lipid-rich spores as an anti-cancer agent with tumour inhibition shown in *in vitro* studies[5-7]. However, a recent comparative study of the immuno-modulatory and anti-tumour activity of the sporoderm-broken spores and whole fruiting body extract showed them to be comparable with no superiority of efficacy for the sporoderm-broken spores[8].

G. lucidum shows exceptionally high tyrosinase inhibition with the highest activity in the aqueous extract. This has led to its inclusion in many commercial skin whitening products and has medical implications, especially in relation to Parkinson's Disease (see discussion under Parkinson's Disease)[9-11].

CANCER - *G. lucidum* has a long history of traditional use in the treatment of cancer and is credited with many cases of spontaneous remission[12,13].

As well as the immune modulating effect of its high polysaccharide content, its triterpenes show significant cytotoxic activity against different cancer cell lines, as well as inhibitory effects against Epstein-Barr virus, known to be associated with some cancers[14-21]. In addition triterpenes from *G. lucidum* show inhibition of the nuclear transcription factor, NF-kappaB (NF-kB), which is overexpressed in various cancer cell lines, and also the AP-1 signalling pathway[22].

Inhibition of NF-kB is of particular importance in the activity of *G. lucidum* against breast and prostate cancers as it is considered to play an essential role in the hormone independent growth and spread of these cancers[23,24].

Studies with *G. lucidum* polysaccharide extract confirm its ability to enhance immune status in cancer patients with increases in NK cell activity and Th1 cytokine levels and decreases in Th2 cytokine levels in advanced lung cancer patients[25,26].

ALLERGIES - As well as immuno-modulatory activity, *G. lucidum* demonstrates strong anti-inflammatory activity with suppression of tumour necrosis factor-alpha (TNF-alpha), interleukin-6 (IL-6), the inflammatory mediator nitric oxide (NO) and prostaglandin E(2), mediated through inhibition of the NF-kB and AP-1 signaling pathways. This combination of immunomodulatory and anti-inflammatory activity contributes to its efficacy in the treatment of allergies and other inflammatory conditions[27-30].

G. lucidum is a component of FAHF-2, a Chinese herbal formula that has been reported to completely block anaphylactic reactions in a mouse model of peanut allergy[31].

LIVER DISEASE - The fruiting body of *G. lucidum* has long been a popular traditional treatment for liver diseases and demonstrates wide hepatoprotective properties[32-36]. It appears that at least part of its action in this regard may be through the ability of *G. lucidum* triterpenes to block platelet-derived growth factor beta receptor (PDGFbetaR), thus inhibiting the activation and proliferation of hepatic stellate cells, a key event in hepatic fibrosis[37].

G. lucidum is also traditionally used in the treatment of hepatitis and in a clinical study of 355 cases of hepatitis B treated with Wulingdan Pill, of which *G. lucidum* is the major component, 92.4% of patients were reported to have positive results[38]. Again, it appears that the triterpenes are the key components[39,40].

HYPERTENSION - *G. lucidum* has a broad range of action on cardiovascular health. Polysaccharides and triterpenes isolated from *G. lucidum* have shown hypolipidemic, hypotensive, and anti-thrombotic effects while a polysaccharide preparation (Ganopoly) led to improved ECG and lowered chest pain, palpitation and shortness of breath in a double-blind, randomized, multi-centre study[41]. Mild ACE-inhibitory activity has also been demonstrated for some of *G. lucidum*'s triterpenoid compounds[42].

INSOMNIA/ANXIETY - The traditional name 'spirit mushroom' points to the sedative action of its triterpenoid components and many herbalists value its benefits in cases of insomnia[43-45]. Christopher Hobbs recommends *G. lucidum* for deficiency insomnia while Mizuno recommends it for 'mental stabilisation'.

RHEUMATOID ARTHRITIS - *G. lucidum*'s combination of immuno-modulatory and anti-inflammatory action suggests potential application in the treatment of autoimmune conditions such as rheumatoid arthritis. A proteoglycan fraction from *G. lucidum* has been shown to inhibit production of rheumatoid arthritis synovial fibroblasts *in vitro*, in part through inhibition of the NF-kB transcription pathway[46].

ANTI-AGING - Traditionally considered to promote longevity, *G. lucidum* extract has been shown to inhibit beta-amyloid synaptic toxicity with potential benefits in Alzheimers Disease[47]. In addition, *G. lucidum*'s broad spectrum cardiovascular, neurological and immune benefits, together with its beneficial effects on blood sugar and cholesterol control[48-51], make it an excellent general health supplement.

CLINICAL SUMMARY

Main Therapeutic Applications - *Allergies, Liver Support, Cancer (especially breast and prostate), Hypertension, Anxiety/Insomnia.*

Together with Cordyceps sinensis, G. lucidum has the most extensive range of indications and combines well with it in treatment of lung and liver conditions, as well as to provide all-round adaptogenic support.

Key Components - *Triterpenes and polysaccharides*

Dose - *Chang reports the daily dose in folk use for cancer as 25-300g/day fruiting body as decoction (aqueous extract)[52], and cases of spontaneous remission have been achieved using similar doses. Concentration ratios of extracts vary with most in the range of 12-18:1. Taking an average concentration ratio of 15:1 this equates to 2-20g/day of extract, with most practitioners using the lower end of the range, in the region of 3-6g/day. For other conditions lower doses in the range of 1-3g /day are usual.*

Levels of both polysaccharides and triterpenes are highest in the fruiting body and are traditionally extracted by hot water decoction (i.e. boiling to make a tea). However, while aqueous extraction is ideal for the polysaccharides, which are highly water soluble, the triterpenes are poorly water-soluble but highly alcohol-soluble. As the polysaccharides are precipitated out of solution by alcohol some manufacturers have taken the step of supplementing polysaccharide-rich aqueous extracts with triterpenes obtained through alcohol extraction in order to combine the benefits of G. lucidum's polysaccharides and triterpenes.

Caution - *Patients on anti-hypertensive and sedative medication. G. lucidum's anti-coagulant properties mean that caution is also required when using it alongside anti-coagulant drugs[53].*

REFERENCES

1. Reishi mushroom: herb of spiritual potency and medical wonder. Willard T. 1990. Pub. Sylvan Press, Issaquah

2. Global marketing of medicinal ling zhi mushroom *Ganoderma lucidum* (W.Curt.:Fr.) Lloyd (Aphyllophoromycetideae) Products and Safety Concerns. Lai T, Gao Y, Zhou S. Int J Med Mushr. 2004;6(2):100

3. *Ganoderma lucidum* and its pharmaceutically active compounds. Boh B, Berovic M, Zhang J, Zhi-Bin L. Biotechnol Annu Rev. 2007;13:265-301

4. *Ganoderma* - a therapeutic fungal biofactory. Paterson R.R. Phytochemistry. 2006;67(18):1985-2001

5. Antitumour activity of the sporoderm-broken germinating spores of *Ganoderma lucidum*. Liu X, Yuan J.P, Chung C.K, Chen X.J. Cancer Lett. 2002;182(2):155-61

6. Sterols and triterpenoids from the spores of *Ganoderma lucidum*. Zhang C.R, Yang S.P, Yue J.M. Nat Prod Res. 2008;22(13):1137-42

7. Chemical constituents of the spores of *Ganoderma lucidum*. Zhang X.Q, Pang G.L, Cheng Y, Wang Y, Ye W.C. Zhong Yao Cai. 2008;31(1):41-4

8. Comparative studies on the immunomodulatory and antitumour activities of the different parts of fruiting body of *Ganoderma lucidum* and *Ganoderma* spores. Yue G.G, Fung K.P, Leung P.C, Lau C.B. Phytother Res. 2008;22(10):1282-91

9. Inhibition of tyrosinase from *Ganoderma lucidum*. Chu H.L, Wu H.C, Yen-Chin Chen Y.C, Kuo J.M. 12th World Food Congress. 2003;166(2):117-20

10. Effects on tyrosinase activity by the extracts of *Ganoderma lucidum* and related mushrooms. Chien C.C, Tsai M.L, Chen C.C, Chang S.J, Tseng C.H. Mycopathologia. 2008;166(2):117-20

11. Dopamine- or L-DOPA-induced neurotoxicity: the role of dopamine quinone formation and tyrosinase in a model of Parkinson's disease. Asanuma M, Miyazaki I, Ogawa N. Neurotox Res. 2003;5(3):165-76

12. Anticancer effects of *Ganoderma lucidum*: a review of scientific evidence. Yuen J.W, Gohel M.D. Nutr Cancer. 2005; 53(1):11-7

13. Regression of gastric large B-Cell lymphoma accompanied by a florid lymphoma-like T-cell reaction: immunomodulatory effect of *Ganoderma lucidum* (Lingzhi)? Cheuk W, Chan J.K, Nuovo G, Chan M.K, Fok M. Int J Surg Pathol. 2007;15(2):180-6

14. Potential of a novel polysaccharide preparation (GLPP) from Anhui-grown *Ganoderma lucidum* in tumour treatment and immunostimulation. Pang X, Chen Z, Gao X, Liu W, Slavin M, Yao W, Yu L.L. J Food Sci. 2007;72(6):S435-42

15. Cytotoxic triterpenoids from *Ganoderma lucidum*. Cheng C.R, Yue Q.X, Wu Z.Y, Song X.Y, Tao S.J, Wu X.H, Xu P.P, Liu X, Guan S.H, Guo D.A. Phytochemistry. 2010;71(13):1579-1585

16. Triterpenes from *Ganoderma lucidum* induce autophagy in colon cancer through the inhibition of p38 mitogen-activated kinase (p38 MAPK). Thyagarajan A, Jedinak A, Nguyen H, Terry C, Baldridge L.A, Jiang J, Sliva D. Nutr Cancer. 2010;62(5):630-40

17. Ganoderic acid T inhibits tumour invasion *in vitro* and *in vivo* through inhibition of MMP expression. Chen N.H, Liu J.W, Zhong J.J. Pharmacol Rep. 2010;62(1):150-63

18. Inhibitory effects of *ganoderma lucidum* on tumourigenesis and metastasis of human hepatoma cells in cells and animal models. Weng C.J, Chau C.F, Yen G.C, Liao J.W, Chen D.H, Chen K.D. J Agric Food Chem. 2009;57(11):5049-57

19. Cytotoxic lanostanoid triterpenes from *Ganoderma lucidum*. Guan S.H, Xia J.M, Yang M, Wang X.M, Liu X, Guo D.A. J Asian Nat Prod Res. 2008;10(7-8):705-10

20. The anti-invasive effect of lucidenic acids isolated from a new *Ganoderma lucidum* strain. Weng C.J, Chau C.F, Chen K.D, Chen D.H, Yen G.C. Mol Nutr Food Res. 2007;51(12):1472-7

21. Lucidenic acids P and Q, methyl lucidenate P, and other triterpenoids from the fungus *Ganoderma lucidum* and their inhibitory effects on Epstein-Barr virus activation. Iwatsuki K, Akihisa T, Tokuda H, Ukiya M, Oshikubo M, Kimura Y, Asano T, Nomura A, Nishino H.J Nat Prod. 2003 Dec;66(12): 1582-5

22. Suppression of the inflammatory response by triterpenes isolated from the mushroom *Ganoderma lucidum*. Dudhgaonkar S, Thyagarajan A, Sliva D.Int Immunopharmacol. 2009;9(11): 1272-80

23. *Ganoderma lucidum* suppresses motility of highly invasive breast and prostate cancer cells. Sliva D, Labarrere C, Slivova V, Sedlak M, Lloyd F.P Jr, Ho N.W. Biochem Biophys Res Commun. 2002;298(4):603-12

24. *Ganoderma lucidum* suppresses growth of breast cancer cells through the inhibition of Akt/NF-kappaB signaling. Jiang J, Slivova V, Harvey K, Valachovicova T, Sliva D. Nutr Cancer. 2004;49(2):209-16

25. Effects of ganopoly (a *Ganoderma lucidum* polysaccharide extract) on the immune functions in advanced-stage cancer patients. Gao Y, Zhou S, Jiang W, Huang M, Dai X. Immunol Invest. 2003;32(3):201-15

26. Effects of water-soluble *Ganoderma lucidum* polysaccharides on the immune functions of patients with advanced lung cancer. Gao Y, Tang W, Dai X, Gao H, Chen G, Ye J, Chan E, Koh H.L, Li X, Zhou S. J Med Food. 2005;8(2):159-68

27. Anti-allergic constituents in the culture medium of *Ganoderma lucidum*. (I). Inhibitory effect of oleic acid on histamine release. Tasaka K, Akagi M, Miyoshi K, Mio M, Makino T. Inflammation Research. 1988;23(3-4):153-6

28. Anti-allergic constituents in the culture medium of *Ganoderma lucidum*. (II). The inhibitory effect of cyclooctasulfur on histamine release. Tasaka K, Mio M, Izushi K, Akagi M, Makino T. Inflammation Research. 1988;23(3-4):157-60

29. Effectiveness of Dp2 nasal therapy for Dp2- induced airway inflammation in mice: using oral *Ganoderma lucidum* as an immunomodulator. Liu Y.H, Tsai C.F, Kao M.C, Lai Y.L, Tsai J.J. J Microbiol Immunol Infect. 2003;36(4):236-428

30. The use of *Ganoderma lucidum* (Reishi) in the management of Histamine-mediated allergic responses. Powell M. Nutritional Practitioner Magazine. October 2004

31. The Chinese herbal medicine formula FAHF-2 completely blocks anaphylactic reactions in murine model of peanut allergy. Srivastava K.D, Kattan J.D, Zou Z.M, Li J.H, Zhang L, Wallenstein S, Goldfarb J, Sampson H.A, Li X.M. J Allergy Clin Immunol. 2005;115(1):171-8

32. Antimutagenic activity of methanolic extract of *Ganoderma lucidum* and its effect on hepatic damage caused by benzo[a]pyrene. Lakshmi B, Ajith T.A, Jose N, Janardhanan K.K. J Ethnopharmacol. 2006;107(2):297-303

33. Effects of *Ganoderma lucidum* polysaccharide on CYP2E1, CYP1A2 and CYP3A activities in BCG-immune hepatic injury in rats. Wang X, Zhao X, Li D, Lou Y.Q, Lin Z.B, Zhang G.L. Biol Pharm Bull. 2007;30(9):1702-6

34. Post-treatment of *Ganoderma lucidum* reduced liver fibrosis induced by thioacetamide in mice. Wu Y.W, Fang H.L, Lin W.C. Phytother Res. 2010;24(4):494-9

35. *In vitro* and *in vivo* protective effects of proteoglycan isolated from mycelia of *Ganoderma lucidum* on carbon tetrachloride-induced liver injury. Yang X.J, Liu J, Ye L.B, Yang F, Ye L, Gao J.R, Wu Z.H. World J Gastroenterol. 2006;12(9):1379-85

36. Antifibrotic effects of a polysaccharide extracted from *Ganoderma lucidum*, glycyrrhizin, and pentoxifylline in rats with cirrhosis induced by biliary obstruction. Park E.J, Ko G, Kim J, Sohn D.H. Biol Pharm Bull. 1997;20(4):417-20.

37. *Ganoderma lucidum* extract attenuates the proliferation of hepatic stellate cells by blocking the PDGF receptor. Wang G.J, Huang Y.J, Chen D.H, Lin Y.L. Phytother Res. 2009;23(6):833-9

38. Treatment of chronic hepatitis B with *Wulingdan Pill*. Journal of the fourth Military Medical College. 8:380-383. From Abstracts of Chinese Medicines 2:188

39. Effects of total Triterpenoids extract from *Ganoderma lucidum* (Curt.: Fr.) P. Karst. (Reishi Mushroom) on experimental liver injury models induced by Carbon Tetrachloride or D-Galactosamine in mice. Lin Z.B, Wang M.Y, Liu Q, Che Q.M. Int J Med Mushr. 2002;4(1):37-41

40. Anti-hepatitis B activities of ganoderic acid from *Ganoderma lucidum*. Li Y.Q, Wang S.F. Biotechnol Lett. 2006;28(11): 837-41

41. A phase I/II study of ling zhi mushroom *Ganoderma lucidum* (W.Curt.:Fr.) Lloyd (*Aphyllophoromycetideae*) extract in patients with coronary heart disease. Gao Y, Chen G, Dai X, Ye J, Zhou S. Int J Med Mushr. 2004;6(4):30

42. Effect of *Ganoderma lucidum* on the quality and functionality of Korean traditional rice wine, yakju. Kim J.H, Lee D.H, Lee S.H, Choi S.Y, Lee J.S. J Biosci Bioeng. 2004;97(1):24-8

43. A preliminary study on the sleep-improvement function of the effective ingredients of *Ganoderma lucidum* fruitbody. Jia W, Wu M, Zhang J.S, Liu Y.F. Acta Edulis Fungi. 2005;12(3):43-47

44. Sleep-promoting effects of *Ganoderma extracts* in rats: comparison between long-term and acute administrations. Honda K, Komoda Y, Inoué S. Tokyo Ika Shika Daigaku Iyo Kizai Kenkyusho Hokoku. 1988;22:77-82

45. Extract of *Ganoderma lucidum* potentiates pentobarbital-induced sleep via a GABAergic mechanis. Chu Q.P, Wang L.E, Cui X.Y, Fu H.Z, Lin Z.B, Lin S.Q, Zhang Y.H. Pharmacology Biochemistry and Behavior 2007;86(4):693-698

46. *Ganoderma lucidum* polysaccharide peptide reduced the production of proinflammatory cytokines in activated rheumatoid synovial fibroblast. Ho Y.W, Yeung J.S, Chiu P.K, Tang W.M, Lin Z.B, Man R.Y, Lau C.S. Mol Cell Biochem. 2007;301(1-2):173-9

47. Antagonizing beta-amyloid peptide neurotoxicity of the anti-aging fungus *Ganoderma lucidum*. Lai C.S, Yu M.S, Yuen W.H, So K.F, Zee S.Y, Chang R.C. Brain Res. 2008;1190:215-24

48. Novel hypoglycemic effects of *Ganoderma lucidum* water-extract in obese/diabetic (+db/+db) mice. Seto S.W, Lam T.Y, Tam H.L, Au A.L, Chan S.W, Wu J.H, Yu P.H, Leung G.P, Ngai S.M, Yeung J.H, Leung P.S, Lee S.M, Kwan Y.W. Phytomedicine. 2009;16(5):426-36

49. Cholesterol-lowering properties of *Ganoderma lucidum in vitro, ex-vivo,* and in hamsters and minipigs. Berger A, Rein D, Kratky E, Monnard I, Hajjaj H, Meirim I, Piguet-Welsch C, Hauser J, Mace K, Niederberger P. Lipids Health Dis. 2004;3:2

50. Ganoderic acid and its derivatives as cholesterol synthesis inhibitors. Komoda Y, Shimizu M, Sonoda Y, Sato Y. Chem Pharm Bull (Tokyo). 1989;37(2):531-3

51. Anti-atherosclerotic properties of higher mushrooms (a clinico-experimental investigation). Li K.R, Vasil'ev A.V, Orekhov A.N, Tertov V.V, Tutel'ian V.A. Vopr Pitan. 1989;(1):16-9

52. Effective dose of *ganoderma* in humans. Chang. In Proceedings of the 5th Int Mycol Congr, Vanvouver. 1994;117-121

53. Experimental and clinical studies on inhibitory effect of *Ganoderma lucidum* on platelet aggregation. Tao J, Feng K.Y. J Tongji Med Univ. 1990;10(4):240-3

Grifola frondosa

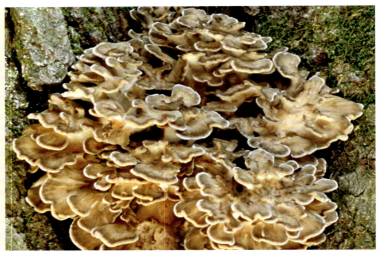

© 2010 Taylor F. Lockwood

Gf

Japanese name
Maitake

Chinese name
Hui Shu Hua

English name
Hen of the Woods

A popular gourmet mushroom, *G. frondosa* is also a highly regarded clinically, especially in cancer therapy.

As with other major anti-cancer mushrooms such as *Lentinus edodes* (Shiitake) and *Trametes versicolor* (Coriolus), polysaccharides have been shown to be the major active components of *G. frondosa* and several beta-glucan, heteropolysaccharide and proteoglycan fractions have been isolated with potent immunomodulatory action, including D-fraction and MD-fraction[1-4].

Most of the clinical research has been carried out by one group of researchers in Japan, initially using D-fraction together with powdered fruiting body, later switching to the more bioactive MD-fraction, again in combination with powdered whole fruiting body.

CANCER - A 1997 paper by Nanba reported benefits from D-fraction taken together with whole fruiting body in a range of stage III-IV cancers with *G. frondosa* increasing the benefit of chemotherapy by an additional 12-28%[5]. The paper further reports synergistic benefits from combining D-fraction and Mitomycin C (MMC) in an animal tumour model with D-fraction (1mg/day) showing superior tumour inhibition to MMC (0.5mg/day) on its own.

A subsequent paper by Nanba et al reported impressive results for MD-fraction and whole *G. frondosa* fruiting body powder in cancer patients who had discontinued chemotherapy because of side effects with improvement in 7 of 12 liver cancer patients, 11 of 16 breast cancer patients and 5 of 8 lung cancer patients, together with increases in IL-2 (a major Th1 cytokine) and CD4+[6].

Further studies confirmed alleviation of side effects from chemotherapy, including loss of appetite, vomiting, nausea, hair loss and leukopaenia, as well as synergy between D-fraction and vitamin C[2,6].

DIABETES - Various animal studies indicate benefit from *G. frondosa* in diabetes models but at high doses, in one case giving 1g/day *G. frondosa* powder to genetically diabetic mice and in another a purified alpha-glucan at a dose of 150-450mg/kg[7,8].

In small scale clinical studies *G. frondosa* polysaccharide extract (dose unknown) was reported to control blood sugar levels in one patient and produce a 30% reduction in blood sugar levels in 4 other patients while inclusion of *G. frondosa* beta-glucans (150mg/day) in yoghurt produced significant improvement in blood glucose levels in 20 type II diabetes patients[3,9].

CHOLESTEROL - Inclusion of *G. frondosa* in the diet of experimental animals at 5-20% of feed produces reductions in cholesterol consistent with the results seen in other mushrooms[10].

HYPERTENSION - A number of studies report short-lived hypotensive action for *G. frondosa* included in the diet of hypertensive animals (typically 5% of feed)[11-13].

CLINICAL SUMMARY

Main Therapeutic Application - *Cancer*

Key Component - *Polysaccharides*

Dose - *The optimum dose of D-fraction/MD-fraction in animal studies is reported to be 1mg/kg i.p. with human trials using D-fraction/MD-fraction at oral doses of 35-150mg/day in combination with 4-6g/day G. frondosa fruiting body.*

REFERENCES

1. A polysaccharide extracted from *Grifola frondosa* enhances the anti-tumour activity of bone marrow-derived dendritic cell-based immunotherapy against murine colon cancer. Masuda Y, Ito K, Konishi M, Nanba H. Cancer Immunol Immunother. 2010
2. Maitake extracts and their therapeutic potential - A review. Mayell M. Alt Med Rev, 2001;6(1)
3. *Grifola frondosa* (Dicks.: Fr.) S.F. Gray (Maitake Mushroom): medicinal properties, active compounds, and biotechnological cultivation. Boh B, Berovic M.M. Int J Med Mushr. 2007;9(2):10
4. Anti tumour activity of orally administered d-fraction from Maitake (*Grifola frondosa*). Nanba H. J Naturopathic Medicine. 1993;1:10-15
5. Maitake D-fraction: healing and preventive potential for cancer. Nanba H. J Orthomolecular Med. 1997;12:43-49
6. Can Maitake MD-fraction aid cancer patients? Kodama N, Komuta K, Nanba H. Alt Med Rev. 2002;(7)3:236-9
7. Anti-diabetic activity present in the fruit body of *Grifola frondosa* (Maitake). Kubo K, Aoki H, Nanba H. Biol Pharm Bull. 1994;17:1106-1110
8. Anti-diabetic effect of an alpha-glucan from fruit body of maitake (*Grifola frondosa*) on KK-Ay mice. Hong L, Xun M, Wutong W. J Pharm Pharmacol. 2007;59(4):575-82
9. Anti-cancer and hypoglycemic effects of Polysaccharides in edible and medicinal Maitake mushroom [*Grifola frondosa* (Dicks.: Fr.) S. F. Gray] Konno S et al. Int J Med Mushr 4:3
10. Anti-hyperliposis effect of Maitake fruit body (*Grifola frondosa*) Kubo K, Nanba H. Biol Pharm Bull. 1997;20:781-785
11. Blood pressure lowering activity present in the fruit body of *Grifola frondosa* (maitake). Adachi K, Nanba H, Otsuka M, Kuroda H. Chen Pharm Bull. 1988;36:1000-1006
12. Effect of shiitake (*Lentinus edodes*) and maitake (*Grifola frondosa*) mushrooms on blood pressure and plasma lipids in spontaneously hypertensive rats. Kabir Y, Yamaguchi M, Kimua S. J Nutr Sci Vitaminol. 1987;33:341-346
13. Dietary mushrooms reduce blood pressure in spontaneously hypertensive rats (SHR). Kabir Y, Kimura S. J Nutr Sci Vitaminol. 1989;35:91-94

Hericium erinaceus

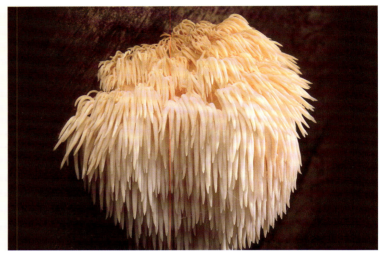

Japanese Name
Yamabushitake

Chinese Name
Hou Tou Gu (Monkey Head Mushroom)

English Name
Lion's Mane Mushroom /Hedgehog Mushroom

© 2010 Taylor F. Lockwood

This delicious mushroom has been referred to as 'Nature's Nutrient for the Neurons' on account of its ability to stimulate the production of nerve growth factor (NGF)[1,2].

NGF plays an essential role in the differentiation and survival of several cell populations in the central and peripheral nervous system and lower than normal levels of NGF have been linked to early stages of both Alzheimers Disease and dementia[3-8].

Although therapeutic interest has largely focussed on its importance for neurological function, NGF plays a much wider role in maintaining homoeostasis in the body[9,10]. It is known to have insulinotropic, angiogenic, and antioxidant properties and reduced plasma levels of NGF have been associated with cardiovascular diseases and metabolic syndromes, including type 2 diabetes[11,12]. It has been shown to accelerate wound healing and there is evidence that it could be useful in the treatment of skin and corneal ulcers[13]. Animal studies have shown NGF to have a profound effect on airway inflammation and asthma-related symptoms with increased NGF levels observed in bronchoalveolar lavage fluid and serum from patients with asthma[14].

NGF also has a dynamic relationship with the immune system. Production of NGF is increased after brain injury, in part due to cytokines produced by immune cells. At the same time cells of the immune system express receptors for NGF, which is involved in immune modulation[15].

Two families of cyathane derivatives from *H. erinaceus* have been identified as being active in the stimulation of NGF production: the hericenones (isolated from the mycelium) and the erinacines (isolated from the fruiting body). Critically these molecules are small enough to pass through the blood-brain barrier. There is also evidence that they can increase myelination[1,16,17].

In China the mycelium is used to make *H. erinaceus* pills to treat gastric and duodenal ulcers, chronic gastritis, gastric and oesophageal cancer.

DEMENTIA - In controlled studies *H. erinaceus* supplementation showed beneficial effects in patients with mild dementia. In one study 6 out of 7 patients showed improvement in functional capacity (understanding, communication, memory etc.) while all 7 showed improved Functional Independence Scores (eating, dressing, walking etc.), after consuming 5g *H. erinaceus* fruiting body daily in soup[1]. In another study, 30 patients aged 50-80 with mild dementia were randomised into treatment and control groups. *H. erinaceus* was given as tablets at 3g/day for 16 weeks and produced significant increases in cognitive function in the treatment group. However, four weeks after the conclusion of the trial, cognitive function scores decreased indicating a need for continued supplementation[17].

MS - *H. erinaceus* fruiting body extract has been shown to improve the myelination process in mature myelinating fibres with possible benefits for MS patients[18,19]. NGF has also been shown to have a protective effect on axons and myelin by suppressing the immune-mediated inflammatory processes responsible for chronic brain destruction in neurodegenerative disorders such as MS by switching the immune response to an anti-inflammatory, suppressive mode in a brain-specific environment[13].

NEUROPATHY - NGF plays a role in pain sensitivity and low NGF levels have been linked to sensory neuropathy in both *in vivo* and *in vitro* studies[10]. Enhanced NGF production has been shown to protect sensory function in diabetic rats and NGF reduction has been shown to cause cardiac sensory neuropathy[21,22].

Clinical studies with recombinant human NGF indicate benefit in patients with diabetic polyneuropathy[23] and NGF has also been reported to reduce pain in patients with HIV associated sensory neuropathy[24,25]. However, ability to promote regeneration of sensory neurons has yet to be demonstrated[26,27].

NERVE DAMAGE - Rats given aqueous extract of *H. erinaceus* fruiting bodies showed faster recovery from nerve injury, suggesting potential for application of *H. erinaceus* in the early stages of nerve regeneration[28].

MRSA - Extracts of both fruiting body and mycelium exhibit anti-MRSA activity with erinacines identified as active compounds. In clinical tests in Japan MRSA is reported to have been cleared in a number of patients whose diet was supplemented with *H. erinaceus*[29].

GASTRITIS - One of the traditional indications for *H. erinaceus*, it appears likely that the antibacterial action of its cyathane derivatives contribute to its action in this regard, with *Helicobacter pylori* now known to be a major cause of chronic gastritis[30-32].

CLINICAL SUMMARY

Main Therapeutic Application - *Dementia, Alzheimers Disease, MS and Nerve Damage.*

Key Component - *Cyathane derivatives including hericenones and erinacines.*

Dose - *Clinical trials support the use of dried fruiting body at a dose of 3-5g/day for increasing NGF production while animal studies on the use of H. erinaceus for gastric ulcers produced the best results with a daily intake of 500mg/kg, which equates to the dosage prescribed in the Chinese Phamacopoeia of 25-50g/day[32,33]. It is likely that similar doses would be required in cases of MRSA[30].*

High in vitro NGF promoting activity of mycelial extracts and the fermentation broth also indicates potential for the use of biomass products[34,35].

Caution - *Asthma and other allergic conditions. Erinacine E is a potent agonist of the kappa opioid receptor with potential hallucinogenic properties[36].*

Long term supplementation

As *H. erinaceus* is a culinary as well as a medicinal mushroom it can be appropriate to incorporate it into the diet for long term supplementation.

Traditional recipes include Hericium Chicken Soup, Hericium Braised Ribs and Hericium Scrambled Eggs! However, these require whole *H. erinaceus*, either fresh or dried, which is rarely available outside China. They also universally recommend soaking the *H. erinaceus* first to remove the bitter principals before cooking, although this is undesirable from a therapeutic perspective.

The best option for most patients is to add 3-5g/day of the more readily available powdered fruiting body to a portion of pre-made soup or stock for a tasty and health-promoting drink (1 tablespoon powdered fruiting body weighs 4.5-5g).

REFERENCES

1. The anti-Dementia effect of Lion's Mane mushroom and its clinical application. Kawagishi H, Zhuang C, Shnidman E. Townsend Letter for Doctors and Patients, 2004
2. Kawagishi H, Shimada A, Hosokawa S, Mori H, Sakamoto H, Ishiguro Y, Sakemi S, Bordner J, Kojima N, Furukawa S. Erinacines E, F, and G, stimulators of nerve growth factor (NGF)-synthesis, from the mycelia of *Hericium erinaceum*. Tetra Lett. 1996 37(41):7399-402
3. Erinacine A increases catecholamine and nerve growth factor content in the central nervous system of rats. M. Shimbo, H. Kawagishi, H. Yokogoshi. Nutrition Research. ;25(6):617-623
4. NGF and BDNF: from nerves to adipose tissue, from neurokines to metabokines. Chaldakov G.N, Tonchev A.B, Aloe L. Riv Psichiatr. 2009;44(2):79-87
5. Development of a non invasive NGF-based therapy for Alzheimer's disease. Covaceuszach S, Capsoni S, Ugolini G, Spirito F, Vignone D, Cattaneo A. Curr Alzheimer Res. 2009;6(2):158-70
6. Neurotrophins: from pathophysiology to treatment in Alzheimer's disease. Schulte-Herbrüggen O, Jockers-Scherübl M.C, Hellweg R. Curr Alzheimer Res. 2008;5(1):38-44

7. One hundred years after the discovery of Alzheimer's disease. A turning point for therapy? Giacobini E, Becker R.E. J Alzheimers Dis. 2007;12(1):37-52

8. Neurotrophic factors—a tool for therapeutic strategies in neurological, neuropsychiatric and neuroimmunological diseases? Schulte-Herbrüggen O, Braun A, Rochlitzer S, Jockers-Scherübl M.C, Hellweg R. Curr Med Chem. 2007;14(22):2318-29

9. Levi-Montalcini R (2004). "The nerve growth factor and the neuroscience chess board". Prog. Brain Res. 146: 525–7

10. Neurotrophin presence in human coronary atherosclerosis and metabolic syndrome: a role for NGF and BDNF in cardiovascular disease?. Prog Brain Res. Chaldakov G.N, Fiore M, Stankulov I.S, Manni L, Hristova M.G, Antonelli A, Ghenev PI, Aloe L. 2004;146:279–89

11. Reduced plasma levels of NGF and BDNF in patients with acute coronary syndromes. Int J Cardiol. Manni L, Nikolova V, Vyagova D, Chaldakov G.N, Aloe L. 2005;102(1):169–71

12. Homo obesus: a metabotrophin-deficient species. Pharmacology and nutrition insight. Curr Pharm Des. Chaldakov G.N, Fiore M, Tonchev A.B, Dimitrov D, Pancheva R, Rancic G, Aloe L. 2007;13(21):2176–9

13. Nerve growth factor and wound healing. Prog Brain Res. Kawamoto K, Matsuda H. 2004;146:369–84

14. Expression of nerve growth factor in the airways and its possible role in asthma. Freund V, Frossard N. Prog Brain Res. 2004;146:335–46

15. Role of nerve growth factor and other trophic factors in brain inflammation". Villoslada P, Genain C.P. Prog Brain Res. 2004;146:403–14

16. Nerve growth factor-inducing activity of *Hericium erinaceus* in 1321N1 human astrocytoma cells. Mori K, Obara Y, Hirota M, Azumi Y, Kinugasa S, Inatomi S, Nakahata N. Biol Pharm Bull. 2008;31(9):1727-32

17. Improving effects of the mushroom Yamabushitake (*Hericium erinaceus*) on mild cognitive impairment: a double-blind placebo-controlled clinical trial. Mori K, Inatomi S, Ouchi K, Azumi Y, Tuchida T. Phytother Res. 2009;23(3):367-72

18. The influence of *Hericium erinaceus* extract on myelination process *in vitro*. Kolotushkina E.V, Moldavan M.G, Voronin K.Y, Skibo G.G. Fiziol Z.H. 2003;49(1):38-45

19. *Hericium erinaceus* (Bull.: Fr.) Pers. extract effect on nerve cells. Grygansky A.P, Moldavan M.G, Kolotushkina O.V, Skibo G.G. Int J Med Mushr. 2001;3(2-3):152

20. Haploinsufficiency of the nerve growth factor beta gene in a 1p13 deleted female child with an insensitivity to pain. Fitzgibbon G.J, Kingston A, Needham M, Gaunt L. Dev Med Child Neurol. 2009;51(10):833-7

21. Protection of sensory function in diabetic rats by Neotrofin. Calcutt N.A, Freshwater J.D, Hauptmann N, Taylor E.M, Mizisin A.P. Eur J Pharmacol. 2006;534(1-3):187-93

22. Nerve growth factor is critical for cardiac sensory innervation and rescues neuropathy in diabetic hearts. Ieda M, Kanazawa H, Ieda Y, Kimura K, Matsumura K, Tomita Y, Yagi T, Onizuka T, Shimoji K, Ogawa S, Makino S, Sano M, Fukuda K. Circulation. 2006;114(22):2351-63

23. Recombinant human nerve growth factor in the treatment of diabetic polyneuropathy. S. C. Apfel et al. Neurology. 1998;51:695-702

24. Long-term treatment with recombinant nerve growth factor for HIV-associated sensory neuropathy. G. Schifitto et al. Neurology. 2001;57:1313-1316

25. A phase II trial of nerve growth factor for sensory neuropathy associated with HIV infection. J. C. McArthur et al. Neurology. 2000;54:1080-1088

26. Regeneration of primary sensory neurons. Donnerer J. Pharmacology. 2003;67(4):169-81

27. Nerve growth factor and diabetic neuropathy. Pittenger G, Vinik A. Exp Diabesity Res. 2003;4(4):271-85

28. Functional recovery enhancement following injury to rodent peroneal nerve by Lion's Mane mushroom, *Hericium erinaceus* (Bull.: Fr.) Pers. (*Aphyllophoromycetideae*). Wong K.H, Naidu M, David R.P, Abdulla M.A, Abdullah N, Kuppusamy U.R, Sabaratnam V. Int J Med Mushr.11(3):20

29. Anti-MRSA compounds of *Hericium erinaceus*. Kawagishi H et al. Int J Med Mushr. 2005;7(3):350

30. A double-blind study of effectiveness of hericium erinaceus pers therapy on chronic atrophic gastritis. A preliminary report. Xu C.P, Liu W.W, Liu F.X, Chen S.S, Liao F.Q, Xu Z, Jiang L.G, Wang C.A, Lu X.H. Chin Med J (Engl). 1985;98(6):455-6

31. Cytoprotective effects of *Hericium erinaceus* on gastric mucosa in rats. Yu C.G, Xu Z.M, Zhu Q.K et al. Chinese J Gastrent. 1999-02

32. Effect of culinary-medicinal Lion's Mane mushroom, *Hericium erinaceus* (Bull.: Fr.) Pers. (*Aphyllophoromycetideae*), on Ethanol-induced gastric ulcers in rats. Abdulla M.A, Noor S, Sabaratnam V, Abdullah N, Wong K.H, Ali H.M. Int J Med Mush. 2008;10(4):325-330

33. Chinese Pharmacopoeia, 2010. Beijing:Chinese Medicine Science and Technology Publishing House

34. Activity of aqueous extracts of Lion's Mane mushroom *Hericium erinaceus* (Bull.: Fr.) Pers. (*Aphyllophoromycetideae*) on the neural cell line NG108-15. Wong K.H, Vikineswary S, Abdullah N, Naidu M, Keynes R. Int J Med Mushr. 2007;9(1):57-65

35. Neurotropic and trophic action of Lion's Mane mushroom *Hericium erinaceus* (Bull.: Fr.) Pers. (*Aphyllophoromycetideae*) extracts on nerve cells *in vitro*. Moldavan M.G, Grygansky A.P, Kolotushkina O.V, Kirchhoff B, Skibo G.G, Pedarzani P. Int J Med Mush. 2007;9(1)

36. Erinacine E as a kappa opioid receptor agonist and its new analogs from a basidiomycete, *Hericium ramosum*. Saito T, Aoki F, Hirai H, Inagaki T, Matsunaga Y, Sakakibara T, Sakemi S, Suzuki Y, Watanabe S, Suga O, Sujaku T, Smogowicz AA, Truesdell SJ, Wong JW, Nagahisa A, Kojima Y, Kojima N. J Antibiot (Tokyo). 1998 Nov;51(11):983-90

Inonotus obliquus

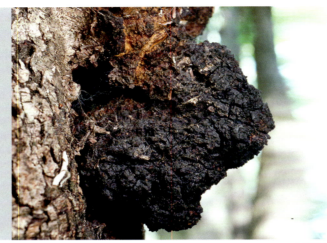

Io

Japanese name
Kabanoanatake

Chinese name
Bai Hua Rong

English name
Chaga

© 2010 Taylor F. Lockwood

I. obliquus grows widely in the forests of Eastern Europe and Russia on several trees, including birch, alder and spruce, where it appears as a sterile growth or conk on the trunk of the tree. The fruiting body is reported to be found growing nearby but is extremely rare in nature.

Traditionally only the *I. obliquus* growing on birch trees was used, as a tea in the treatment of cancers including inoperable breast cancer, hip, gastric, parotid, pulmonary, stomach, skin, rectal and Hodgkins disease[1] and *I. obliquus* is recorded as a miraculous cure for cancer in Solzhenitsyn's semi-autobiographical 1967 novel, the 'Cancer Ward'.

The wisdom of using birch grown *I. obliquus* is supported by the finding that one of its key components is the triterpene betulinic acid, which occurs naturally in a number of plants but primarily in the bark of the white birch (*Betula pubescens* - seen as the tree of life and fertility in many Eastern European and Siberian myths) from which it gets its name. *I. obliquus* growing on the birch trees takes up high concentrations of betulinic acid from the bark of the trees, making it and its derivatives available in an absorbable form.

Betulinic acid has been shown to induce mitochondrial apoptosis in different cancer cell lines and inhibit the enzyme topoisomerase[2], which is essential for the unwinding and winding of the DNA strands in cell replication. In addition it possesses anti-retroviral, anti-parasitic and anti-inflammatory properties[3]. It is currently being developed as an anti-cancer agent through the Rapid Access to Intervention Development program of the US National Cancer Institute and is also a major contributor to the anti-cancer action of mistletoe[4].

Other important components of *I. obliquus* include polysaccharides and sterols. Its high phenolic content gives it exceptional antioxidant properties and a melanin complex has also been identified as having significant antioxidant and genoprotective properties[5,6].

CANCER - Widely used in Poland and Russia as a folk remedy against cancer[7], *I. obliquus* is now attracting increasing interest among practitioners with its combination of immune supporting polysaccharides and components with direct anti-cancer activity, especially betulinic acid derivatives.

In vitro studies on betulinic acid have shown it to be highly effective against a wide variety of cancer cells: human melanoma, neuroectodermal (neuroblastoma, medulloblastoma, Ewing's sarcoma) and malignant brain tumours, ovarian cancer, human leukaemia HL-60 cells and malignant head and neck squamous cell cancers, including those derived from therapy-resistant and refractory tumours[8,9]. However, it was found to have no effect on epithelial tumours, such as breast cancer, colon cancer, small cell lung cancer and renal cell cancer as well as T-cell leukaemia cells. Its anti-tumour activity has been related to its direct effects on mitochondria and induction of apoptosis, irrespective of cells p53 status[10].

Clinically betulinic acid's action against brain cancer cells is particularly interesting and it is noteworthy that in one study it exerted cytotoxic activity against primary tumour cells cultured from patients in 4 of 4 medulloblastoma-tumour samples tested and in 20 of 24 glioblastoma-tumour samples[11]. It also shows great promise in combination with radiotherapy, exhibiting a strictly additive mode of growth inhibition in combination with radiation in human melanoma cells in one study and acting as a radiosensitizer in head and neck squamous cell cancers in another[12,13].

In vivo studies confirm its anti-cancer action as well as a complete absence of systemic toxicity in rodents[8].

ANTI-VIRAL - *I. obliquus* has traditionally been used to treat a number of viral conditions and betulinic acid analogs have been shown to disrupt assembly and budding of the HIV-1 virus and viral fusion to the cell membrane[9].

CLINICAL SUMMARY

Main Therapeutic Applications - *Cancer, Anti-viral, antioxidant*

Key Component - *Betulinic acid derivatives*

Dose - *It is reported that only aqueous extracts prepared by boiling, as done traditionally, show anti-tumour activity[14]. Recommended dosage for aqueous extract as powder is 2-5g/day.*

REFERENCES

1. Plants used against cancer. Hartwell J.L. 1982. Quartermain Pubs: Lawrence, Mass. p.694
2. Betulinic acid, a potent inhibitor of eukaryotic topoisomerase I: identification of the inhibitory step, the major functional group responsible and development of more potent derivatives. Chowdhury A.R, Mandal S, Mittra B, Sharma S, Mukhopadhyay S, Majumder H.K. Medical Science Monitor. 2002;8(7):254–65
3. Antimalarial activity of betulinic acid and derivatives *in vitro* against *Plasmodium falciparum* and *in vivo* in *P. berghei*-infected mice. de Sá M.S, Costa J.F, Krettli A.U, Zalis M.G, Maia G.L,

Sette I.M, Câmara Cde A, Filho J.M, Giulietti-Harley A.M, Ribeiro Dos Santos R, Soares M.B. Parasitol Res. 2009;105(1):275-9

4. Solubility studies of oleanolic acid and betulinic acid in aqueous solutions and plant extracts of *Viscum album* L. Jäger S, Winkler K, Pfüller U, Scheffler A. Planta Med. 2007;73(2):157-62

5. Antioxidant small phenolic ingredients in *Inonotus obliquus* (persoon) Pilat (Chaga). Nakajima Y, Sato Y, Konishi T. Chem Pharm Bull (Tokyo). 2007;55(8):1222-6

6. Melanin complex from medicinal mushroom *Inonotus obliquus* (Pers.: Fr.) Pilat (Chaga) (*Aphyllophoromycetideae*). Bisko N.A, Mitropolskaya N.Y, Ikonnikova N.V. Int J Med Mushr. 2002;4(2):139-145

7. Study of anticarcinogenic properties of *Poria obliqua* Patalog. Nazarewicz T, Konopa J. Pol. 1961;1:80-82

8. Betulinic acid, a natural compound with potent anticancer effects. Mullauer F.B, Kessler J.H, Medema J.P. Anticancer Drugs. 2010;21(3):215-27. 2010;24(1):90-114

9. Betulinic acid induces apoptosis in human neuroblastoma cell lines. Schmidt M.L, Kuzmanoff K.L, Ling-Indeck L, Pezzuto J.M. European Journal of Cancer. 1997;33(12):2007–10

10. Chemistry, biological activity, and chemotherapeutic potential of betulinic acid for the prevention and treatment of cancer and HIV infection. Cichewicz R.H, Kouzi S.A. Med Res Rev. 2004;24(1): 90-114

11. Betulinic acid: a new cytotoxic agent against malignant brain-tumour cells. Fulda S, Jeremias I, Steiner H.H, Pietsch T, Debatin K.M. Int J Cancer. 1999;82(3):435-41

12. Effects of betulinic acid alone and in combination with irradiation in human melanoma cells. Selzer E, Pimentel E, Wacheck V, et al. The Journal of Investigative Dermatology. 2000;114(5):935–40

13. Betulinic acid - a radiosensitizer in head and neck Squamous cell carcinoma cell lines. Eder-Czembirek C, Erovic B.M, Czembirek C, Brunner M, Selzer E, Pötter R, Thurnher D. Strahlenther Onkol. 2010

14. Medicinal Mushrooms. An exploration of tradition, healing and culture. Hobbs C. 1986. Pub Botanica Press, Williams

Lentinus edodes
(Lentinula edodes)

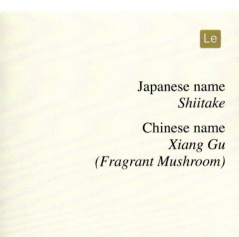

Le

Japanese name
Shiitake

Chinese name
Xiang Gu
(*Fragrant Mushroom*)

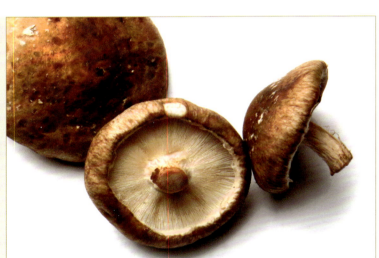

L. edodes is an important ingredient in Asian cuisine and its annual production (2 million tons) is second only to the common button mushroom (*Agaricus bisporus*). As well as being delicious, it has an excellent nutritional profile with high levels of B vitamins and pro-vitamin D2 (ergosterol)[1].

LEM, a crude mycelial extract from *L. edodes* with proven immuno-modulating properties contains glycoproteins, nucleic acid derivatives, vitamin B compounds and ergosterol while Lentinan, a highly purified polysaccharide from *L. edodes*, is licensed in Japan for the treatment of gastric cancer.

Other bioactive compounds from *L. edodes* include eritadenine, which shows promise for lowering cholesterol levels, and Lentin, an anti-fungal protein which also inhibits HIV-1 reverse transcriptase activity and proliferation of leukaemia cells[2].

Uniquely among the medicinal mushrooms high levels of consumption have been reported to cause an allergic skin reaction termed Shiitake Dermatitis and although there are no reports of reactions at supplementation levels caution or an alternative choice of mushroom are advised in those with sensitive skin[3,4].

CANCER - Analysis of 5 clinical trials with a total of 650 participants shows that the addition of Lentinan at 2mg/week to standard chemotherapy offers a significant advantage over chemotherapy alone in terms of survival for patients with advanced gastric cancer, patients with lymph node metastasis having slightly better results than patients without[5].

Additional trials confirm increased survival, reduced side effects from chemotherapy and improved quality of life in patients with colorectal, hepatocelluar, breast cancer and metastatic prostate cancer[6]. In a trial with 69 metastatic prostate cancer patients the 50% survival length of treated and control patients was 48 and 35 months respectively, while the five-year survival rate of treated patients was 43% against 29% in the control group[7].

Although usually delivered by injection, Lentinan is also orally bioavailable although the clinical dosage is likely to be significantly higher [8,9].

CHOLESTEROL CONTROL - Eritadenine has been shown to be a potent inhibitor of S-adenosylhomocysteine hydrolase and to accelerate excretion of ingested cholesterol and its metabolic decomposition. When added to the diet of rats (0.005%), eritadenine caused a 25% decrease in total cholesterol in one week[1].

Early studies indicated that levels found in whole shiitake mushrooms were too small to have a significant effect but recent research has shown the presence of eritadenine at levels 10 times higher than originally, indicating therapeutic possibilities for shiitake, particularly in cases where patients have shown statin intolerance[10,11].

In clinical trials dried *L. edodes* (9g/day) decreased serum cholesterol 7-10% in patients suffering from hypercholesterolemia and 90g/day fresh *L. edodes* (equivalent to 9g/day dried mushroom) led to a decrease in total cholesterol of 9-12% and triglycerides of 6-7%[1].

HEPATITIS B - Polysaccharides extracts from *L. edodes* have been shown to be hepato-protective and in a study of 40 patients with chronic hepatitis B, LEM at 6g/day for 4 months led to improved liver function and resulted in 17 patients becoming seronegative for Hbe antigen (HbeAg)[1,9].

HIV - LEM increased the T-cell count in HIV patients with AIDS symptoms from 1250/mm^3 to 2550/mm^3 after 60 days[1].

CANDIDA - *In vitro* studies show *L. edodes* to have consistently high levels of anti-microbial activity, including the highest anti-candidal action among several mushroom species (for further discussion see section on Candidiasis).

CLINICAL SUMMARY

Main Therapeutic Application - *Cancer, cholesterol control, especially as an adjunct to statins*

Key Components - *Polysaccharides and eritadenine*

Dose - *2-6g/day polysaccharide extract for immune support. 9g/day dried fruit body for cholesterol control.*

Because eritadenine's cholesterol lowering action differs from that of prescription statins or natural sources of statins such as Pleurotus ostreatus or Monascus purpureus, it can usefully be combined with them in cholesterol control protocols.

Caution - *Patients with sensitive skin.*

REFERENCES

1. Shiitake (*Lentinus edodes*) Wasser SP. Encyclopedia of Dietary Supplements. 2005
2. Lentin, a novel and potent antifungal protein from shitake mushroom with inhibitory effects on activity of human immunodeficiency virus-1 reverse transcriptase and proliferation of leukaemia cells. Ngai P.H, Ng T.B. Life Sci. 2003;73(26): 3363-74
3. Shiitake dermatitis now occurs in France. Hérault M, Waton J, Bursztejn A.C, Schmutz J.L, Barbaud A. Ann Dermatol Venereol. 2010;137(4):290-3
4. Shiitake dermatitis: flagellate dermatitis after eating mushrooms. Hautarzt. Haas N, Vogt R, Sterry W. 2001;52(2):132-5
5. Individual patient based meta-analysis of lentinan for unresectable /recurrent gastric cancer. Oba K, Kobayashi M, Matsui T, Kodera Y, Sakamoto J. Anticancer Res. 2009;29(7):2739-45
6. Effects of lentinan in advanced or recurrent cases of gastric, colorectal, and breast cancer. Taguchi T. Gan To Kagaku Ryoho. 1983;10(2 Pt 2):387-93
7. Effect of lentinan for advanced prostate carcinoma. Tari K, Satake I, Nakagomi K, Ozawa K, Oowada F, Higashi Y, Negishi T, Yamada T, Saito H, Yoshida K. Hinyokika Kiyo. 1994;40(2): 119-23
8. Inhibition of human colon carcinoma development by lentinan from shiitake mushrooms (*Lentinus edodes*). Ng M.L, Yap A.T. J Altern Complement Med. 2002;8(5):581-9
9. The medicinal benefits of Lentinan (β-1, 3-D glucan) from *Lentinus edodes* (Berk.) singer (Shiitake Mushroom) through oral administration. Yap A.T, Ng M.H. Int J Med Mushr. 2005;7(12):170
10. Production of the bioactive compound eritadenine by submerged cultivation of shiitake (*Lentinus edodes*) mycelia. Enman J, Hodge D, Berglund K.A, Rova U. J Agric Food Chem. 2008;56(8):2609-12
11. Quantification of the bioactive compound eritadenine in selected strains of shiitake mushroom (*Lentinus edodes*). Enman J, Rova U, Berglund K.A. J Agric Food Chem. 2007;55(4):1177-80
12. Shiitake, *Lentinus edodes*: Functional properties for medicinal and food purposes Mizuno T. Food Reviews International, 1995;1(1):109-128

Phellinus linteus

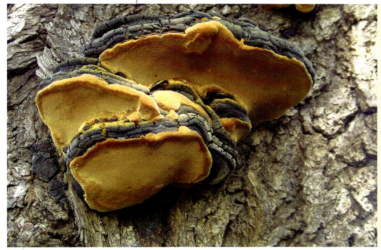

© 2010 Dr Frankie Chan

Japanese name
Meshimakobu

Chinese name
Sang Huang
(Mulberry Yellow)

P. linteus is a basidiomycete fungus, popular in China, Korea and Japan and reported to work as a 'miracle medicine', prolonging longevity. Identified by Ikekawa as having the highest anti-tumour activity of the Hymenomycetes[1] (a fungal grouping containing the major medicinal mushrooms), and by Stamets as having the greatest macrophage activation of 7 species surveyed[2], it has been heavily researched in the last decade, especially in Korea, showing broad immunostimulant activity, strong anti-cancer properties and the ability to enhance the efficacy of existing chemotherapeutic drugs[3].

Uniquely among the medicinal mushrooms, the Chinese Pharmacopoeia describes the energy of *P. linteus* as Cold (see section on Medicinal Mushrooms According to Traditional Chinese Medicine) and ascribes to it an extensive range of indications, including: cancer, diabetes, HIV, angina, leucorrhoea, diarrhoea and accelerated wound healing.

Research has focussed on *P. linteus*' polysaccharide and proteoglycan components.

CANCER - Interest in the potential of *P. linteus* in cancer therapy has been stimulated by recent reports of remarkable effects in a number of cancer patients taking it. One case reported dramatic remission in a case of hormone refractory prostate cancer with rapidly progressive bone metastasis[4], while in a second a 65 year old man with a large hepatocellular cancer and metastasis in the skull, sternum and ribs, who declined all treatment except radiation for the painful frontal bone mass in favour of *P. linteus*, experienced spontaneous regression of the tumours[5]. In a third case spontaneous regression of hepatocellular cancer with multiple lung metastasis was linked to consumption of *P. linteus* mycelium (no conventional therapy undertaken)[6].

In vitro studies show that low levels of *P. linteus* polysaccharides induce cell cycle arrest in lung cancer cells[7] and exhibit synergistic action with chemotherapeutic drugs such as doxorubicin, inducing apoptosis at a sub-therapeutic dose in prostate and lung cancer cells[8], while at high doses activating apoptosis in lung cancer cells, hormone sensitive and, to a lesser degree, refractory prostate cancer cells, as well as suppressing growth, angiogenesis and invasive behaviour of breast cancer cells[9,10]. Modes of action identified include inhibition of Akt signalling and caspase induction.

In vitro studies also show significant inhibition of bladder cancer cell growth with enhanced cytotoxic activity in combination with vitamin C[11].

In vivo studies show significantly prolonged survival, reduced tumour growth and reduced frequency of lung metastasis in mice transplanted with melanoma cells after administration of polysaccharide extract[12,13].

RHEUMATOID ARTHRITIS - In a murine rheumatoid arthritis model polysaccharide extract from *P. linteus* fruiting bodies reduced expression of pro-inflammatory Th2 cytokines (such as TNF-α and IFN-γ) and increased expression of anti-inflammatory Th1 cytokines, including IL-10 and TGF-β, resulting in the subsidence of the auto-immune response in the joints of the mice. Similar results were seen with polysaccharides from the related species *Phellinus rimosus*[14,15].

P. linteus polysaccharides have also been shown to reduce expression of TNF-α and major histocompatability complex II expression in lipopolysaccharide induced septic shock, supporting their use as anti-inflammatory agents[16].

ALLERGIES - Several studies show strong effect of *P. linteus* polysaccharides in suppressing production of Th2 cytkines and promoting secretion of Th1 cytokines, thereby addressing the immune imbalance involved in allergic responses[17-19]. At the same time it is reported that aqueous extract of *P. linteus* fruiting body prevented histamine release in response to allergenic stimuli and inhibited mast cell mediated anaphylaxis-like reactions[20,21].

CLINICAL SUMMARY

Therapeutic Application - *Cancer, rheumatoid arthritis, allergies*

Key Component - *Polysaccharides*

Dose - *The Chinese Pharmacopoeia prescribes a daily dose of 10-30g for the dried mushroom, while for polysaccharide extract 2-5g/day is usual*[22].

REFERENCES

1. Antitumour activity of some basidiomycetes, especially *Phellinus linteus*. Ikekawa et al. Jpn J Cancer Res. 1968;59:155-157
2. Potentiation of cell-mediated host defense using fruitbodies and mycelia of medicinal mushrooms. Stamets P. Int J Med Mushr. 2003;5:179-191
3. A medicinal mushroom: *Phellinus linteus*. Zhu T, Kim S.H, Chen C.Y. Curr Med Chem. 2008;15(13):1330-5
4. Dramatic remission of hormone refractory prostate cancer achieved with extract of the mushroom, *Phellinus linteus*. Shibata Y, Kurita S, Okugi H, Yamanaka H. Urol Int. 2004;73(2):188-90
5. Spontaneous regression of a large hepatocellular carcinoma with skull metastasis. Nam S.W, Han J.Y, Kim J.I, Park S.H, Cho S.H, Han N.I, Yang J.M, Kim J.K, Choi S.W, Lee Y.S, Chung K.W, Sun H.S. J Gastroenterol Hepatol. 2005;20(3):488-92
6. A case of spontaneous regression of hepatocellular carcinoma with multiple lung metastases. Kojima H, Tanigawa N, Kariya S, Komemushi A, Shomura Y, Sawada S, Arai E, Yokota Y. Radiat Med. 2006;24(2):139-42
7. Modulation of lung cancer growth arrest and apoptosis by *Phellinus Linteus*. Guo J, Zhu T, Collins L, Xiao Z.X, Kim S.H, Chen C.Y. Mol Carcinog. 2007;46(2):144-54
8. *Phellinus linteus* sensitises apoptosis induced by doxorubicin in prostate cancer. Collins L, Zhu T, Guo J, Xiao Z.J, Chen C.Y. Br J Cancer. 2006;95(3):282-8
9. *Phellinus linteus* activates different pathways to induce apoptosis in prostate cancer cells. Zhu T, Guo J, Collins L, Kelly J, Xiao Z.J, Kim S.H, Chen C.Y. Br J Cancer. 2007;96(4):583-90
10. *Phellinus linteus* suppresses growth, angiogenesis and invasive behaviour of breast cancer cells through the inhibition of AKT signalling. Sliva D, Jedinak A, Kawasaki J, Harvey K, Slivova V. Br J Cancer. 2008;98(8):1348-56
11. Effect of various natural products on growth of bladder cancer cells: two promising mushroom extracts. Konno S, Alt Med Rev. 2007;12(1):63-68
12. Acidic polysaccharide from *Phellinus linteus* inhibits melanoma cell metastasis by blocking cell adhesion and invasion. Han S.B, Lee C.W, Kang J.S, Yoon Y.D, Lee K.H, Lee K, Park S.K, Kim H.M. Int Immunopharmacol. 2006;6(4):697-702
13. The inhibitory effect of polysaccharide isolated from *Phellinus linteus* on tumour growth and metastasis. Han B, Lee C.W, Jeon Y.J, Hong N.D, Yoo I.D, Yang K.H, Kim H.M. Immunopharmacology. 1999;41:157-164
14. Oral administration of proteoglycan isolated from *Phellinus linteus* in the prevention and treatment of collagen-induced arthritis in mice. Kim G.Y, Kim S.H, Hwang S.Y, Kim H.Y, Park Y.M, Park S.K, Lee M.K, Lee S.H, Lee T.H, Lee J.D. Biol Pharm Bull. 2003;26(6):823-31
15. Antiarthritic activity of a Polysaccharide-protein complex isolated from *Phellinus rimosus* (Berk.) Pilát (*Aphyllophoromycetideae*) in Freund's complete adjuvant–induced arthritic rats. Meera C.R, Smina T.P, Nitha B, Mathew J, Janardhanan K.K. Int J Med Mushr. 2009;11(1):21-28
16. Alleviation of experimental septic shock in mice by acidic polysaccharide isolated from the medicinal mushroom *Phellinus linteus*. Kim G.Y, Roh S.I, Park S.K, Ahn S.C, Oh Y.H, Lee J.D, Park Y.M. Biol Pharm Bull. 2003;26(10):1418-23
17. Stimulation of humoral and cell mediated immunity by polysaccharide from mushroom *Phellinus linteus*. Kim H.M, Han S.B, Oh G.T, Kim Y.H, Hong D.H, Hong N.D, Yoo I.D. Int J Immunopharmac. 1996;18(5):295-303
18. *Phellinus linteus* extract augments the immune response in Mitomycin C-induced immunodeficient mice. Matsuba S, Matsuno H, Sakuma M, Komatsu Y. Evid Based Complement Alternat Med. 2008;5(1):85-90.6
19. *Phellinus linteus* grown on germinated brown rice suppresses IgE production by the modulation of Th1/Th2 balance in murine mesenteric lymph node lymphocytes. Lim B.O, Jeon T.I, Hwang S.G, Moon J.H, Park D.K. Biotechnol Lett. 2005;27(9):613-7
20. Inhibition of anaphylaxis-like reaction and mast cell activation by water extract from the fruiting body of *Phellinus linteus*. Choi Y.H, Yan G.H, Chai O.H, Lim J.M, Sung S.Y, Zhang X, Kim J.H, Choi S.H, Lee M.S, Han E.H, Kim H.T, Song C.H. Biol Pharm Bull. 2006;29(7):1360-5
21. Inhibitory effects of *Agaricus blazei* on mast cell-mediated anaphylaxis-like reactions. Choi Y.H, Yan G.H, Chai O.H, Choi Y.H, Zhang X, Lim J.M, Kim J.H, Lee M.S, Han E.H, Kim H.T, Song C.H. Biol Pharm Bull. 2006;29(7):1366-71
22. Chinese Pharmacopoeia, 2010. Beijing:Chinese Medicine Science and Technology Publishing House

Pleurotus ostreatus

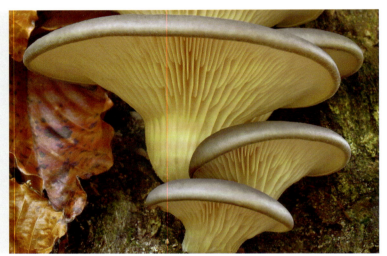

English name
Oyster Mushroom

Chinese name
Ping Gu

Japanese name
Hiratake

© 2010 Jaroslav Malý

One of the principal culinary mushrooms, *P. ostreatus* fruiting bodies contain lovastatin in concentrations ranging from 0.7-2.8% dried weight depending on the strain.

P. ostreatus has also been commercialized as a source of beta-glucans and related polysaccharides for immune support and shows promise as an anti-aging dietary supplement.

CHOLESTEROL CONTROL - Dried *P. ostreatus* fed to hamsters at 2% of a high fat diet for 6 months is reported to have lowered VLDL by 65-80% and total serum lipid levels by 40% and to totally negate increases in triglyceride and liver cholesterol levels associated with chronic alcohol intake[1-3]. Multiple animal studies show *P. ostreatus* fed at 5% of diet to produce improvements in blood lipid levels[4-10]. Intake of more than 5% was seen to suppress appetite[11].

Bobek et al report reductions in cholesterol in humans from intake of 15-20g/day[5] and in a small 'proof of concept' study, 20 HIV patients taking protease inhibitors who had elevated non-HDL cholesterol (>160mg/dl) were given 15g/day freeze-dried *P. ostreatus* for 8 weeks resulting in an increase of HDL from an average of 37 to 40.2mg/dl and a decrease in triglycerides from 320.5 to 271.3 but no significant reduction in non-HDL cholesterol[12] (abnormalities in lipid metabolism are a common side effect of anti-retroviral treatment). Khatun et al also reported *P. ostreatus* to reduce cholesterol levels in diabetic patients[13].

ANTI-AGING - As well as having immunomodulatory, anti-cancer and hepatoprotective properties in common with those from other mushrooms, polysaccharides from *P. ostreatus* have been shown to increase activity of catalase, superoxide dismutase and glutathione peroxidase, as well as counter age-related reductions in levels of vitamins C and E [14-19].

CLINICAL SUMMARY

Therapeutic Application - *General health maintenance, especially in the elderly. Can be prescribed for cholesterol control, although Monascus purpureus products (Hong Qu Mi - Red Yeast Rice) usually give a more controlled dose of lovastatin*

Key Components - *Lovastatin, polysaccharides*

Dose - *For general health maintenance 2-3g/day polysaccharide extract. For cholesterol control 10-15g/day dried fruit body.*

Caution - *Patients taking protease inhibitors such as ritonavir, indinavir etc., which have been shown to raise statin levels significantly through common use of the CYP3A4 enzyme system.*

REFERENCES

1. Effect of mushroom *Pleurotus ostreatus* and isolated fungal polysaccharide on serum and liver lipids in Syrian hamsters with hyperlipoproteinemia. Bobek P, Ginter E, Kuniak L, Babala J, Jurcovicova M, Ozdín L, Cerven J. Nutrition. 1991;7(2):105-8
2. Cholesterol-lowering effect of the mushroom *Pleurotus ostreatus* in hereditary hypercholesterolemic rats. Bobek P, Ginter E, Jurcovicová M, Kuniak L. Ann Nutr Metab. 1991;35(4):191-5
3. Effect of oyster fungus (*Pleurotus ostreatus*) on serum and liver lipids of Syrian hamsters with a chronic alcohol intake. Bobek P, Ginter E, Jurcovicová M, Ozdín L, Mekinová D. Physiol Res. 1991;40(3):327-32
4. Dose-dependent hypocholesterolaemic effect of oyster mushroom (*Pleurotus ostreatus*) in rats. Bobek P, Ozdín L, Kajaba I. Physiol Res. 1997;46(4):327-9
5. Dose- and time-dependent hypocholesterolemic effect of oyster mushroom (*Pleurotus ostreatus*) in rats. Bobek P, Ozdín L, Galbavý S. Nutrition. 1998;14(3):282-6
6. Hypocholesterolic activity of the genus *Pleurotus* (Jacq.: Fr.) P. Kumm. (*Agaricales s. I., Basidiomycetes*) Nina Gunde-Cimerman et al, Int J Med Mushr 2001;3(4)
7. Evidence for the anti-hyperlipidaemic activity of the edible fungus *Pleurotus ostreatus*. Opletal L, Jahodár L, Chobot V, Zdanský P, Lukes J, Brátová M, Solichová D, Blunden G, Dacke C.G, Patel A.V. Br J Biomed Sci. 1997;54(4):240-3
8. Dietary mushroom (*Pleurotus ostreatus*) ameliorates atherogenic lipid in hypercholesterolaemic rats. Hossain S, Hashimoto M, Choudhury E.K, Alam N, Hussain S, Hasan M, Choudhury S.K, Mahmud I. Clin Exp Pharmacol Physiol. 2003;30(7):470-5
9. Role of oyster mushroom (*Pleurotus florida*) as hypocholesterolemic/antiatherogenic agent. Bajaj M, Vadhera S, Brar A.P, Soni G.L. Indian J Exp Biol. 1997;35(10):1070-5
10. Cholesterol-lowering effect of Pleurotus species (*Agaricomycetideae*) (Abstracts of papers published in 1991-1999) Bobek P. Int J Med Mushr. 1999;1(4):371-380
11. A lectin from the edible and medicinal mushroom *Pleurotus ostreatus* (Jacq.: Fr.) Kumm. as a food intake suppressing substance. Yokoyama S, Nakamura H, Tokuyama S. Int J Med Mush. 2001;3(2-3)
12. Antihyperlipidemic effect of *Pleurotus ostreatus* in HIV: results of a pilot proof-of-principle clinical trial. Abrams D.I, Couey P, Shade S.B, Kelly M.E, Kamanu-Elias N, Stamets P.E. Int J Med Mushr. 2007;9(3):204
13. Oyster mushroom reduced blood glucose and cholesterol in diabetic subjects. Khatun K, et al Mymensingh Med J. 2007;16(1):94-9
14. Effect of oyster mushroom (*Pleurotus ostreatus*) on pathological changes in dimethylhydrazine-induced rat colon cancer. Bobek P, Galbavy S, Ozdin L. Oncol Rep. 1998;5(3):727-30
15. Cytotoxic effect of oyster mushroom *Pleurotus ostreatus* on human Androgen-independent prostate cancer PC-3 cell. Gu Y.H, Sivam G. J Med Food. 2006;9(2):196-204
16. Effects of *Lentinus edodes, Grifola frondosa* and *Pleurotus ostreatus* administration on cancer outbreak and activities of macrophages and lymphocytes in mice treated with a carcinogen N-butyl-N-butnolnitrosamine. Kurashige S, Aleusawa Y, Endo F. Immunopharm. Immunodetox. 1997;19:175-183
17. Antioxidant activity of the oyster mushroom, *Pleurotus ostreatus*, on CCl(4)-induced liver injury in rats. Jayakumar T, Ramesh E, Geraldine P. Food Chem Toxicol. 2006;44(12):1989-96
18. Protective effect of an extract of the oyster mushroom, *Pleurotus ostreatus*, on antioxidants of major organs of aged rats. Jayakumar T et al. Exp Gerontol. 2007;42(3):183-91
19. An extract of the oyster mushroom, *Pleurotus ostreatus*, increases catalase gene expression and reduces protein oxidation during aging in rats. Thanasekaran J, Aloysius P.T, Mathivanan I, Pitchairaj G.J. Chin Int Med. 2010;8(8):774-780

Polyporus umbellatus
(Grifola umbellata)

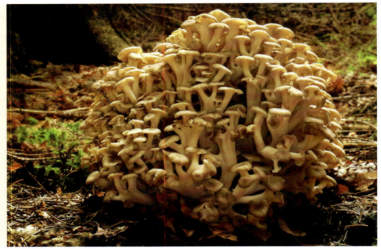

Chinese Name
Zhu Ling
(sclerotium)

Japanese Name
Chorei Maitake
(fruiting body)

© 2010 Gerhard Schuster

A close relative of *Grifola frondosa* (Maitake), *P. umbellatus* differs from most medicinal mushrooms in that traditionally it has been harvested as a hyphal mass, or sclerotium, which only forms when *P. umbellatus* is symbiotically associated with Armillaria species[1,2].

Li Shi Zhen, in his comprehensive materia medica the *Ben Cao Gang Mu* (1578), says of this mushroom's actions, quoting the earlier *Shen Nong Ben Cao*, 'dispersing invading vicious factors and facilitating urination. Long term use makes one feel happy and vigorous and look younger'[3].

As well as its traditional use as a diuretic, polysaccharide extracts of *P. umbellatus* show promise as adjuvant nutrition alongside chemotherapy and are licensed in China for use in cancer therapy[4]. A number of steroids with cytotoxic activity against cancer cells have also been isolated from the fruiting body[5-7].

DIURETIC - *P. umbellatus* is a component of the classical diuretic herbal formula *Wu Ling San* and a number of compounds have been identified as contributing to its diuretic activity, including triterpenes, ergosterol and d-mannitol[8-10].

Comparison with other diuretics, including *Poria cocos* and caffeine, indicates that *P. umbellatus* has stronger action with oral administration of 8g aqueous decoction leading to a 62% increase in 6-hour urine output and a 54.5% increase in chloride excretion[4].

CANCER - Co-administration of *P. umbellatus* polysaccharide extracts with chemotherapy is reported to improve treatment outcomes and quality of life indicators in patients with a number of cancers including lung, liver, leukaemia, nose and throat[11-13].

In vivo studies confirm increases in survival when given with chemotherapy (119.9% compared to 70.1% for Mitomycin C on its own in experimental liver cancer[12]) and *in vitro* and *in vivo* studies show broad effects on the immune system, including TLR4 mediated macrophage activation and increased antibody production[11,15,16].

P. umbellatus aqueous extract significantly inhibited the development of bladder cancer in rats exposed to N-butyl-N-(4-hydroxybutyl) nitrosamine, with 61.1% of animals in the treatment group developing cancer compared to 100% in the control group, and it was also reported to be effective in reducing recurrence in 22 patients with recurrent bladder cancer[17,18].

In addition *P. umbellatus* polysaccharides prevented the development of toxohormone-L (a compound produced by cancer cells) induced cachexia (loss of weight, muscle atrophy, fatigue) in rats[19], while a number of steroids from *P. umbellatus* show promise as agents for promoting hair regrowth with low doses of extract (1.28 and 6.4 μg/ml) found to markedly enhance hair growth and lengthen the period of hair growth[20].

CLINICAL SUMMARY

Therapeutic Application - *Cancer, fluid retention*

Key Component - *Polysaccharides*

Dose - *While the sclerotium has traditionally been prescribed as a diuretic in formulae at a dose of 6-15g/day, polysaccharide extracts are preferred for cancer care - 3-6g/day polysaccharide extract.*

Caution - *Patients on prescription diuretics.*

REFERENCES

1. Involvement of Ca2+ Channel Signalling in Sclerotial Formation of *Polyporus umbellatus*. Ying-Ying Liu and Shun-Xing Guo. Mycopathologia. 2009;169(2):139-150
2. Identification of Armillaria species associated with *Polyporus umbellatus* using ITS sequences of nuclear ribosomal DNA. Gen Kikuchi and Hiroki Yamaji. Mycoscience. 2010;51(5):366-372
3. Compendium of Materia Medica (Ben Cao Gang Mu). Li Shi Zhen. Tran. Luo Xiwen. 2003. Beijing:Foreign Languages Press
4. Pharmacology and Applications of Chinese Materia Medica. Chang H.M, But P.P.H. 1986. Singapore:World Scientific
5. Studies on constituents of fruit body of *Polyporus umbellatus* and their cytotoxic activity. Ohsawa T, Yukawa M, Takao C, Murayama M, Bando H. Chem Pharm Bull (Tokyo). 1992;40(1):143-7
6. Cytotoxic steroids from *Polyporus umbellatus*. Zhao Y.Y, Chao X, Zhang Y, Lin R.C, Sun W.J. Planta Med. 2010
7. Simultaneous determination of eight major steroids from *Polyporus umbellatus* by high-performance liquid chromatography coupled with mass spectrometry detections. Zhao Y.Y, Cheng X.L, Zhang Y, Zhao Y, Lin R.C, Sun W.J. Biomed Chromatogr. 2010;24(2):222-30
8. Bioactivity-directed isolation, identification of diuretic compounds from *Polyporus umbellatus*. Zhao Y.Y, Xie R.M, Chao X, Zhang Y, Lin RC, Sun W.J. J Ethnopharmacol. 2009;126(1):184-7
9. An anti-aldosteronic diuretic component (drain dampness) in *Polyporus sclerotium*. Yuan D, et al. Biol Pharm Bull. 2004;27(6):867-70
10. Diuretic activity and kidney medulla AQP1, AQP2, AQP3, V(2)R expression of the aqueous extract of sclerotia of *Polyporus umbellatus* FRIES in normal rats. Zhang G, Zeng X, Han L, Wei J.A, Huang H. J Ethnopharmacol. 2010

11. Recent advances on the active components in Chinese medicine. Zhu D. Abstracts of Chinese Medicines. 1987;1:251-286
12. Review on the studies of antineoplastic fungal polysaccharides. Li M. Jiangxi Zhongyiyao. 1985;63:59-61
13. Chinese Medical Herbology and Pharmacology. Chen J.K, Chen T.T. 2001:386. Pub. Art of Medicine Press, City of Industry
14. Combined effects of chuling (*Polyporus umbellatus*) extract and mitomycin C on experimental liver cancer. You J.S, Hau D.M, Chen K.T, Huang H.F. Am J Chin Med. 1994;22(1):19-28
15. TLR4-mediated activation of macrophages by the polysaccharide fraction from *Polyporus umbellatus*(pers.) Fries. Li X, Xu W. J Ethnopharmacol. 2010
16. Polysaccharide purified from *Polyporus umbellatus* (Per) Fr induces the activation and maturation of murine bone-derived dendritic cells via toll-like receptor 4. Li X, Xu W, Chen J. Cell Immunol. 2010;265(1):50-6
17. Inhibitory effect of Chinese herb medicine zhuling on urinary bladder cancer. An experimental and clinical study. Yang D.A. Zhonghua Wai Ke Za Zhi. 1991;29(6):393-5,399
18. Prevention of postoperative recurrence of bladder cancer: a clinical study. Yang D, Li S, Wang H, Li X, Liu S, Han W, Hao J, Zhang H. Zhonghua Wai Ke Za Zhi. 1999;37(8):464-5
19. Inhibitive effect of *umbellatus polyporus* polysaccharide on cachexic manifestation induced by toxohormone-L in rats. Wu G.S, Zhang L.Y, Okuda H. Zhongguo Zhong Xi Yi Jie He Za Zhi. 1997;17(4):232-3
20. Studies of the active substances in herbs used for hair treatment. II. Isolation of hair regrowth substances, acetosyringone and polyporusterone A and B, from *Polyporus umbellatus* Fries. Ishida H, Inaoka Y, Shibatani J, Fukushima M, Tsuji K. Biol Pharm Bull. 1999;22(11):1189-92

Poria cocos

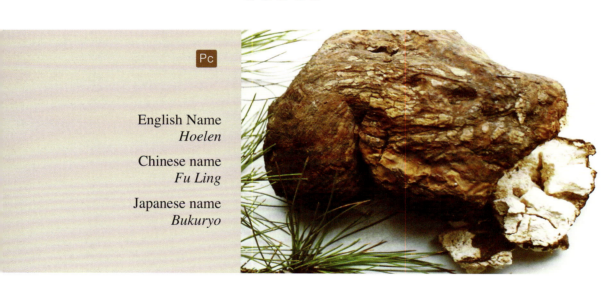

Pc

English Name
Hoelen

Chinese name
Fu Ling

Japanese name
Bukuryo

P. cocos is a component in many traditional Chinese herbal formulae, with functions described as diuretic, tonic and sedative, but is almost never used singly. As the fruiting body is rarely seen, *P. cocos*, like *Polyporus umbellatus,* is traditionally harvested as the sclerotium from the roots of the pine trees on which it grows.

Research has focused on two fractions: polysaccharides and triterpenes, with the triterpenes showing wider activity. Although the majority of the the sclerotium (91-98%) is composed of polysacharides the vast majority are insoluble and most evidence suggests that, unlike in mushrooms such as *P. umbellatus* and *Grifola frondosa*, the soluble polysaccharides have low immunological activity.

CANCER - Triterpenes and heteropolysaccharides from *P. cocos* both show anti-tumour activity[1]. Triterpenes isolated from the sclerotium exhibited inhibitory effects on skin tumour promotion in mice[2-4].

ANTI-INFLAMMATORY - Triterpene fractions from *P. cocos* show strong anti-inflammatory activity in animal models of dermatitis, suppressing carrageenan, arachidonic acid, tetradecanoyl phorbol acetate (TPA) acute oedemas, TPA chronic inflammation and oxazolone delayed hypersensitivity in mice. The fact that triterpenes are found primarily in the outer portion of the poria supports the traditional use of this part for treating inflammatory conditions[5,6,7,8].

ANTI-EMETIC - Triterpenes isolated from *P. cocos* showed anti-emetic activity in frogs[9].

CLINICAL SUMMARY

Main Therapeutic Application - *Mainly used in Chinese herbal formulae to reinforce/balance the effects of other herbs*

Key Components - *Triterpenes*

Dose - *9-15g/day dried herb is used traditionally in aqueous decoctions. However, for single use the tincture is preferred in order to enhance extraction of the triterpenes.*

REFERENCES

1. Antitumour activities of heteropolysaccharides of *Poria cocos* mycelia from different strains. Jin Y, Zhang L, Zhang M, Chen L, Keung P.C, Cheung, Oi V.E.C, Lin Y. Carbohydrate Research. 2003;338(14):1517-1521

2. Triterpene acids from *Poria cocos* and their anti-tumour-promoting effects. Akihisa T, et al J Nat Prod. 2007;70(6):948-53

3. Anti-tumour-promoting effects of 25-methoxyporicoic acid A and other triterpene acids from *Poria cocos*. Akihisa T, Uchiyama E, Kikuchi T, Tokuda H, Suzuki T, Kimura Y. J Nat Prod. 2009;72(10):1786-92

4. Inhibition of tumour-promoting effects by poricoic acids G and H and other lanostane-type triterpenes and cytotoxic activity of poricoic acids A and G from *Poria cocos*. Ukiya M, Akihisa T, Tokuda H, Hirano M, Oshikubo M, Nobukuni Y, Kimura Y, Tai T, Kondo S, Nishino H. J Nat Prod. 2002;65(4):462-5

5. Isolation of inhibitors of TPA-induced mouse ear edema from Hoelen, *Poria cocos*. Nukaya H, Yamashiro H, Fukazawa H, Ishida H, Tsuji K. Chem Pharm Bull (Tokyo). 1996;44(4):847-9

6. Effect of the basidiomycete *Poria cocos* on experimental dermatitis and other inflammatory conditions. Cuellar M.J, Giner R.M, Recio M.C, Just M.J, Mañez S, Rios J.L.Chem Pharm Bull (Tokyo). 1997;45(3):492-4

7. 3β-p-Hydroxybenzoyldehydrotumulosic acid from *Poria cocos*, and its anti-inflammatory effect. Yasukawa K, Kaminaga T, Kitanaka S, Tai T, Nunoura Y, Natori A, Takido M. Phytochemistry. 1998;48(8):1357-1360

8. Antioxidant activity of anti-inflammatory plant extracts. Schinella G.R, Tournier H.A, Prieto J.M, Mordujovich de Buschiazzo P, Ríos J.L. Life Sciences. 2002;70(9):1023-1033

9. Anti-emetic principles of *Poria cocos*. Tai T, Akita Y, Kinoshita K, Koyama K, Takahashi K, Watanabe K. Planta Med 1995;61(6):527-530

Trametes versicolor
(Coriolus versicolor)

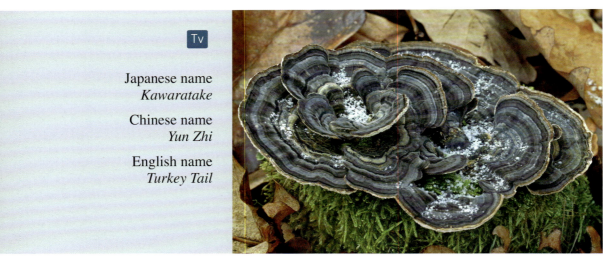

Japanese name
Kawaratake

Chinese name
Yun Zhi

English name
Turkey Tail

© 2010 Jaroslav Malý

T. versicolor is the most extensively researched of all the medicinal mushrooms with large scale clinical trials on the extracts: PSK ('Krestin') and PSP in a variety of cancers, including gastric, oesophageal, lung, breast and colorectal, showing impressive results [1-8].

PSK and PSP are both polysaccharide-protein complexes that are soluble in water but insoluble in ethanol[9]. PSK contains 34-35% polysaccharide (~92% glucan) and 28-35% protein[10].

PSK has been shown to boost immune cell production, ameliorate chemotherapy and radiotherapy side effects, enhance immune status and tumour infiltration by dendritic and cytotoxic cells and significantly extend survival in cancers of the stomach, colon-rectum, oesophagus, nasopharynx, uterus and lung (non-small cell types), and in an HLA B40-positive breast cancer subset in combination with conventional treatment[1]. In addition to its immune related effects, PSK has shown an ability to enhance superoxide dismutase and glutathione peroxidase activity[11,12].

PSP has been shown to significantly enhance immune status in 70-97% of patients with cancers of the stomach, oesophagus, lung, ovary and cervix[8].

Although most clinical trials have been conducted with the above proteoglycan extracts, there is also evidence of immunomodulatory action for *T. versicolor* biomass, with improvements of immune status in patients with chronic fatigue syndrome and enhanced clearance of low grade squamous intraepithelial lesions (LSIL) from the cervix.

CANCER - As mentioned above, the use of *T. versicolor* extracts in cancer treatment is supported by an impressive level of clinical evidence[8]:

STOMACH CANCER - Multiple clinical trials of PSK given alongside surgery and chemotherapy at 3-6g/day significantly extended survival times in stomach cancer at all stages. Even in patients with advanced stomach cancer with metastasis PSK doubled 2 year and 5 year survival and extended 15-year survival.

COLORECTAL - In different clinical trials PSK extended 5-year and 8-year survival after surgery and chemotherapy and after surgery, chemotherapy and radiotherapy.

LUNG CANCER (NSCLC) **STAGES I-III** - PSK extended 5-year survival 2-4x for all cancer stages with stage III cancer patients taking PSK having a better prognosis than stage II patients without PSK.

OESOPHAGEAL - PSK extended 5-year survival after surgery, radiotherapy and chemotherapy while in double-blind trials PSP significantly extended five-year survival in oesophageal cancer as well as improving quality of life, providing substantial pain relief and enhancing immune status in 70-97 percent of patients with cancers of the stomach, oesophagus, lung, ovary and cervix at a dose of 3g/day.

NASOPHARYNGEAL - PSK extended 5-year survival but not disease-free period after radiotherapy and chemotherapy.

BREAST CANCER - Evidence from clinical trials (given alongside chemotherapy) is mixed. In one trial PSK was shown to extend survival in patients with oestrogen receptor negative, non-metastasised, stage II cancer but no benefit was shown in another. In a third trial significant benefit was seen in patients positive for HLA B40 with 100% survival after 10 years.

CERVICAL/UTERINE CANCER - In combination with radiotherapy PSK (3-6g/day) given to patients with stage III uterine and cervical cancer enhanced survival and increased sensitivity of the cancers to radiotherapy. In another trial cervical cancer patients given the same dose together with radiotherapy showed clearance of cancer cells in 36% of patients versus 11% of controls and improved 5-year survival from 48% to 79%. In a recent study using *T. versicolor* biomass, supplementation with 3g/day produced a 72.5% regression rate in LSIL lesions, compared to 47.5% without supplementation, and also increased the clearance of high risk HPV strains from 8.5% to 91.5%[13].

HIV - In several *in vitro* experiments PSK was found to exhibit anti-HIV activity through multiple routes[9,14,15]:

- Inhibition of HIV reverse transcriptase
- Inhibition of viral binding to lymphocytes
- Inhibition of cell-to-cell infection of HIV-1 and HIV-2

Use of *T. versicolor* supplementation (3.0g/day *T. versicolor* biomass) has been reported to improve HIV patients' immune status and produce improvement in HIV related Kaposi's sarcoma[16,17].

HERPES - Clinically *T. versicolor* supplementation is seen to reduce the frequency of Herpes simplex virus (HSV) outbreaks and it has also been shown to inactivate HSV in a dose-dependent manner[18].

CHRONIC FATIGUE SYNDROME (ME) - *T. versicolor* biomass has shown promise in the treatment of Chronic Fatigue Syndrome with immune system activation and increased NK cell activity reported in patients at 1.5g/day (3.0/day for the first 2 weeks) over a 2 month period[19].

HEPATOPROTECTIVE - *T. versicolor* polysaccharide extracts demonstrate hepatoprotective properties[20,21].

CLINICAL SUMMARY

Main Therapeutic Application - *Cancer*

Key Component - *Polysaccharides*

Dose - *Commercial polysaccharide extracts are commonly prescribed at 3g/day and dosage for crude polysaccharide extracts is typically 3-6g/day for cancer and 1-2g/day for immune support. For chronic immune deficient conditions the biomass shows promise at 3g/day, while biomass products have also been used for cancer treatment at 15g/day.*

REFERENCES

1. Krestin (PSK). Tsukagoshi S, Hashimoto Y, Fujii G, Kobayashi H, Nomoto K, Orita K. Cancer Treat Rev. 1984;11(2):131-55
2. Anticancer effects and mechanisms of polysaccharide-K (PSK): Implications of cancer immunotherapy. Fisher M, Yang L.X. Anticancer Res. 2002;22:1737-1754
3. A review of research on the protein-bound polysaccharide (polysaccharopeptide, PSP) from the mushroom *Coriolus versicolor* (Basidiomycetes: Polyporaceae). Ng T.B. Gen Pharmacol. 1998;30(1):1-4
4. Polysaccharopeptides of *Coriolus versicolor*: physiological activity, uses, and production. Cui J, Chisti Y. Biotechnol Adv. 2003;21(2):109-22
5. Effects of PSK on T and dendritic cells differentiation in gastric or colorectal cancer patients. Kanazawa M, Yoshihara K, Abe H, Iwadate M, Watanabe K, Suzuki S, Endoh Y, Takita K, Sekikawa K, Takenoshita S, Ogata T, Ohto H. Anticancer Res. 2005;25(1B):443-9
6. The immunomodulator PSK induces *in vitro* cytotoxic activity in tumour cell lines via arrest of cell cycle and induction of apoptosis. Jiménez-Medina E, Berruguilla E, Romero I, Algarra I, Collado A, Garrido F, Garcia-Lora A. BMC Cancer. 2008;8:78
7. *Trametes versicolor* mushroom immune therapy in breast cancer. Standish L.J, Wenner C.A, Sweet E.S, Bridge C, Nelson A, Martzen M, Novack J, Torkelson C. J Soc Integr Oncol. 2008;6(3):122-8
8. The use of mushroom glucans and proteoglycans in cancer treatment. Parris K. Alternative Medicine Rev. 2000:5(1)
9. Medicinal value of turkey tail fungus *Trametes versicolor* (L.:Fr.) Pilát (*Aphyllophoromycetideae*). A Literature Review. Christopher Hobbs. Int J Med Mushr 2004;6(3)
10. Method of producing nitrogen-containing polysaccharides. Ueno S, Yoshikumi C, Hirose F, Omura Y, Wada T, Fujii T et al. 1980. US Patent 4,202,969

11. Polysaccharide Krestin enhances manganese superoxide dismutase activity and mRNA expression in mouse peritoneal macrophages. Pang Z.J, Chen Y, Zhou M. Am J Chin Med. 2000;28:331-341
12. Effect of polysaccharide krestin on glutathione peroxidase gene expression in mouse peritoneal macrophages. Pang Z.J, Chen Y, Zhou M. Brit J Biomed. 2000;57:130-16
13. *Coriolus versicolor* supplementation in HPV patients. Couto S., da Silva D.P. 20th European Congress of Obstetrics and Gynaecology, 2008
14. A biological response modifier, PSK, inhibits reverse transcriptase *in vitro*. Hirose K, Hakozaki M, Kakuchi J, Matsunaga K, Yoshikumi C, Takahashi M, Tochikura T.S, Yamamoto N. Biochem Biophys Res Commun. 1987;149(2):562-7
15. Polysaccharopeptide from the turkey tail fungus *Trametes versicolor* (L.:Fr.) Pilát inhibits human immunodeficiency virus type 1 reverse Transcriptase and Protease. Tzi Bun Ng, Hexiang Wang, Wan D. C. C. Int J Med Mushr. 2006;8(1):39-43
16. The clinical use of *Coriolus versicolor* supplementation in HIV+ patients and the impact on CD4 count and viral load. Pfeiffer M. 3rd International Symposium on Mushroom Nutrition, 2001
17. The effectiveness of *Coriolus versicolor* supplementation in the treatment of Kaposi sarcoma in HIV+Patients. Tindall J, Clegg E. 10th International Congress of Mucosal Immunology, 1999
18. *in vitro* inactivation of herpes simplex virus by a biological response modifier, PSK. Monma Y, Kawana T, Shimizu F. Antiviral Res. 1997;35:131-138
19. Coriolus. Jean Munroe. J Integrative Medicine. 2004;8:101-108
20. Effects of a hot water extract of *Trametes versicolor* on the recovery of rat liver function. Kim B.K et al. Int J Med Mushr. 2000;2(1):35-42
21. Pharmacological studies on certain mushrooms from china. Ooi V.E.C. Int J Med Mushr. 2001;3(4):341-354

Tremella fuciformis

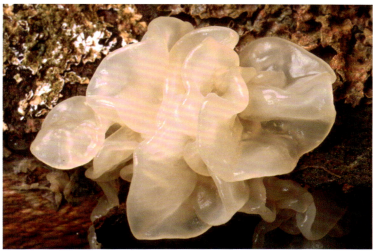

© 2010 Taylor F. Lockwood

English name
Snow Fungus

Japanese name
Shirokikurage / Hakumokuji

Chinese name
Bai Mu Er/Yin Er

As well as being a popular culinary mushroom in oriental cuisine, *T. fuciformis* has a long history of medicinal use and was one of the mushrooms included in the *Shen Nong Ben Cao* (c.200AD). Its traditional indications include clearing heat and dryness, nourishing the brain and enhancing beauty!

Like other jelly fungi, *T. fuciformis* is rich in polysaccharides and these are the main bioactive component[1]. The principal polysaccharide is a glucoronoxylomannan with a linear backbone of 1,3 linked α-D-mannan residues with side chains consisting mainly of xylose and glucoronic acid[2,3]. The glucuronic acid side chains in *Auricularia auricula* have been found to be essential for its anti-coagulant action and they are likely to contribute to *T. fuciformis*'s action in this regard. Unlike in some other mushrooms research has shown no effect on immunological activity from changes in size of the polysaccharide molecules[2].

Research in China has focused on its use to alleviate the side effects of radiotherapy and as an anti-aging supplement with over 40 Chinese patents citing it during the 1990's alone[4,5].

RADIOTHERAPY - As well as demonstrating broad immuno-modulatory activity and *in vitro* anti-cancer activity[6-8], *T. fuciformis* polysaccharides have been shown to protect against the consequences of acute radiation exposure, restoring the blood-producing mechanism of the bone marrow[9]. When administered at a dose of 200mg/kg for 3-5 days prior to Cobalt-60 irradiation they exerted a protective effect on bone marrow with myeloid granulocytes reduced to 60% of normal with *T. fuciformis* polysaccharides but 20% of normal without[10]. They also significantly increased 30-day survival rates in mice, dogs and monkeys exposed to Cobalt-60 γ-rays[11].

CIRCULATORY DISORDERS - *T. fuciformis* polysaccharides have been shown to stimulate DNA synthesis in vascular endothelial cells, the dysfunction of which is a major factor in the pathogenesis of atherosclerosis, hypertension and thrombophlebitis, with therapeutic implications for these conditions. They have also been shown to protect endothelium cells from histamine damage, increase clotting time, reduce platelet adherence and blood viscosity[9].

NEUROLOGICAL DAMAGE - The water extract of *T. fuciformis* (0.01-1 microg/ml) promoted neurite outgrowth of PC12 cells in a dose dependent manner, indicating potential for application of *T. fuciformis* polysaccharides in the treatment of neurological damage[12].

Experiments with mice also showed the ability of *T. fuciformis* polysaccharides to exert an anti-aging effect by increasing the superoxide dismutase activity of the brain and liver[9].

MEMORY IMPAIRMENT - Traditionally considered to nourish the brain, supplementation with *T. fuciformis* polysaccharide extract (100 or 400 mg/kg) for 14 days significantly reversed the scopolamine-induced deficit in learning and memory in rats and alleviated decrease in cholinergic immuno-reactivity induced by scopolamine in the medial septum and hippocampus.

COSMETIC APPLICATION - As mentioned above, *T. fuciformis* has traditionally been used to benefit the skin and 'enhance beauty' and *T. fuciformis* polysaccharides have been developed for use in cosmetics on account of their excellent skin moisture retention, skin protection, flexibility and flattening effects, as well as anti-inflammatory and anti-allergenic properties. Their ability to prevent senile degeneration of micro-vessels also helps maintain blood perfusion to the skin[13].

CLINICAL SUMMARY

Main Therapeutic Application - *Immune support, anti-aging, radiotherapy*

Key Component - *Polysaccharides*

Dose - *1-3g/day polysaccharide extract for health maintenance, 3-6g/day for radiotherapy support.*

T. fuciformis polysaccharides are beneficial for counteracting the harmful effects of radiotherapy and also possess excellent anti-aging activity with a combination of neurological, circulatory and immune-modulating benefits. In addition they are an ideal supplement for those who smoke because of their moistening and nourishing properties, as well as beneficial effects on the skin and immune system.

Caution - *Patients on anti-coagulant medication.*

REFERENCES

1. Research advances in primary biological effects of *Tremella* polysaccharides. Chen FF, Cai DL. Zhong Xi Yi Jie He Xue Bao. 2008;6(8):862-6
2. Characterisation of acidic heteroglycans from *Tremella fuciformis* Berk with cytokine stimulating activity. Gao Q, Seljelid R, Chen H, Jiang R. Carbohydrate Research. 1996;288:135-142
3. Antioxidation activities of polysaccharides extracted from *Tremella fuciformis* Berk. Liu P, Gao X, Xu W, Zhou Z, Shen X. Chinese Journal of Biochemical Pharmaceutics. 2005;03
4. Effect of polysaccharides from *Auricularia auricula* underw, *Tremella fuciformis* Berk and spores of *Tremella fuciformis* Berk on aging. Chen Yi-jun et al. Chinese Journal of Modern Applied Pharmacy. 1989-02
5. Effect of *Tremella* polysaccharides on the immune function of experimental aging model mice. La Y, Liu X, Pei S, Shi Y, Cai D. Chinese Journal of Clinical Nutrition. 2005-04
6. Effect of *Tremella* polysaccharide on IL-2 production by mouse splenocytes. Ma L, Lin Z.B. Yao Xue Xue Bao. 1992;27(1):1-4
7. Effects of *Tremella* polysaccharides on immune function in mice. Xia D, Lin Z.B. Zhongguo Yao Li Xue Bao. 1989;10(5):453-7
8. Antitumour activity on sarcoma 180 of the polysaccharides from *Tremella fuciformis* Berk. Ukai S, Hirose K, Kiho T, Hara C, Irikura T. Chem Pharm Bull (Tokyo). 1972;20(10):2293-4
9. Medicinal value of the genus *Tremella* Pers. (Heterobasidiomycetes) (Review). Reshetnikov S.V, Wasser S.P, Duckman I, and Tsukor K. 2000. Int J Med Mushr. 2000;2:345-367
10. Effect of nourishing Yin and antitoxic capsule II on oxidative injury by X-ray irradiation in rats. Chen R, Shi H.J, Hou Y. Journal of Hebei Medical University. 2006-05
11. Effect of *Tremella fuciformis* Berk on acute radiation sickness in dogs. Zhao T.F, Xu C.X, Li Z.W, Xie F, Zhao Y.T, Wang S.Q, Luo C.H, Lu R.S, Ni G.L, Ku Z.Q, Ni Y.F, Qian Q, Chen X.Q. Zhongguo Yi Xue Ke Xue Yuan Xue Bao. 1982;4(1):20-3
12. Effect of *Tremella fuciformis* on the neurite outgrowth of PC12h cells and the improvement of memory in rats. Kim J.H, Ha H.C, Lee M.S, Kang J.I, Kim H.S, Lee S.Y, Pyun K.H, Shim I. Biol Pharm Bull. 2007;30(4):708-14
13. *Tremella fuciformis* (Shirokikurage) polysaccharide. Ahashi Y, Yamamoto Y. Fragrance Journal. 2005;33,3:45-50

Medicinal Mushrooms in Cancer Therapy

Cancer has traditionally been one of the main conditions for which medicinal mushrooms have been used and in the Far East several mushroom extracts are licensed as adjuvant nutrition for cancer therapy, including:

- PSK and PSP - Proteoglycan extracts from *Trametes versicolor* mycelium
- Lentinan - Polysaccharide extract from *Lentinus edodes* fruit body
- Schizophyllan - Polysaccharide extract from *Schizophyllan commune* culture broth

These extracts have impressive risk/benefit profiles with large scale clinical trials demonstrating extended survival times in a range of cancers and a complete absence of serious side effects[1].

Medicinal mushrooms' broad range of immunological effects (see Introduction) make them ideally suited for support in cases of cancer, with the ability to:

- Facilitate a more effective immune response to the cancer
- Increase tumour cell apoptosis and inhibit tumour growth and metastasis
- Increase the efficacy and reduce the side-effects of conventional treatment

Medicinal Mushrooms and Chemotherapy

Mushroom extracts, such as PSK and PSP, are routinely prescribed alongside a range of chemotherapeutic agents, including cyclophosphamide, Camptothecin, Mitomycin C and 5-Fluorouracil, reducing the side effects of chemotherapy, including nausea, hair loss and lowered immune status, as well improving appetite, general condition and haematopoietic parameters[2-10].

Many other mushroom extracts have shown synergistic activity with chemotherapeutic drugs including:

- Lentinan extended survival in inoperable or recurrent gastric cancer in conjunction the tegafur with a 50% survival time of 173 days compared to 92 days with tegafur alone[11]. Lentinan has also been shown to inhibit Th2 activity and increase Cytotoxic T-cell activity in the spleen when administered to gastric cancer patients undergoing chemotherapy.
- *Armillaria mellea* polysaccharide protected mice bone marrow cells from damage by cyclophosphamide[12].

- *Hericium erinaceus* enhanced doxorubicin-induced apoptosis in liver cancer cells[13].
- *Ganoderma lucidum* triterpenes enhanced doxorubicin-induced apoptosis in HeLa (cervical cancer) cells and prevented cisplatin-induced nephrotoxicity[14,15].
- *Grifola frondosa* polysaccharide fractions potentiated the action of carmustine and increased efficacy when given in combination with chemotherapy across a range of cancers, as well as reducing cisplatin-induced nephrotoxicity[16].
- A hot-water extract of *Cordyceps sinensis* significantly enhanced recovery from taxol-induced leukopenia in mice[17].
- Polysaccharide extract from *S. commune* enhanced recovery of cellular immunity after chemotherapy[18,19].

It appears likely that, as well as supporting the immune system and ameliorating the immune suppression induced by chemotherapy, mushroom polysaccharide extracts may also contribute to the efficacy of the chemotherapeutic drugs themselves through enhanced production of reactive oxygen species (ROS).

Liu et al reported an increase in ROS and reactive nitrogen intermediates in peritoneal macrophages of mice given PSP[20], and Grifron-D, a polysaccharide extract from *Grifola frondosa*, has been shown to have a direct cytotoxic effect on cancer cells through oxidative membrane damage leading to apoptosis[21].

Although mushrooms also show antioxidant activity, this is strongly correlated with pro-oxidant activity, as well as with their respective polysaccharide and polyphenol content, indicating that possible excess cell defense-related intracellular ROS generated by mushroom extracts may be downregulated by the antioxidant components present in the same extracts[22].

CLINICAL NOTE

Medicinal mushrooms may offer some protection against venous thromboembolism (VTE), which some chemotherapy drugs are known to increase the risk of (the annual incidence of VTE in patients receiving chemotherapy is estimated at 11% and this can climb to 20% or higher depending on the type of drug(s) being administered)[23]. Elderly patients are especially at risk and mushrooms with anti-coagulant properties (such as G. lucidum and Tremella fuciformis) can be useful in such cases.

Caution - *Because of medicinal mushrooms' ability to support immune function in patients receiving chemotherapy, they are contraindicated with immunosuppressive chemotherapy for autoimmune conditions.*

Medicinal Mushrooms and Radiotherapy

As with chemotherapy, evidence for synergistic benefit between medicinal mushrooms and radiotherapy is widespread, including:

- *Tremella fuciformis* polysaccharide extract markedly improved the recovery rate of hemopoiesis in irradiated mice, with increased nucleated cells in the bone-marrow, and endogenous colonies in the spleen, without apparent effect on cell radio-sensitivity. In a trial with 136 patients undergoing radiotherapy, oral consumption of *T. fuciformis* polysaccharide extract (3g/day) resulted in a 13.2% reduction in WBC compared to a 35.2% reduction in the control group[24,25]. Other experiments on dogs and monkeys confirm the benefits of *T. fuciformis* polysaccharides in protecting against the effects of Cobalt-60 radiation[26].

- PSP in combination with radiotherapy significantly increased the percentage of apoptotic cells at 24hr compared to radiation alone and reduced radiotherapy induced reduction in white blood cell count[27].

- *Trametes versicolor* biomass (6g/day) prevented decreases in red and white blood cells in lung cancer patients undergoing radiotherapy[28].

- Hot water extract from *Cordyceps sinensis* protected mice from radiation-induced bone marrow and intestinal damage[29].

Medicinal Mushrooms and Surgery

Mushroom extracts such as PSK and Lentinan are routinely used alongside surgical excision of tumours with no contraindication. In addition, two double-blind placebo-controlled studies at Harvard Medical School showed beta-glucan (2g/day) to be effective at protecting patients from infection after undergoing major surgery, indicating their role in enhancing host immunity[1,2].

CLINICAL NOTE

Mushrooms with anti-coagulant properties are best avoided immediately before surgery. The main mushrooms in this category are Antrodia camphorata, Auricularia auricula, Ganoderma lucidum and Tremella fuciformis.

Research on Medicinal Mushrooms in Cancer

Bladder Cancer Pu

Clinical studies in China showed polysaccharide extracts of *Polyporus umbellatus* to be as effective in preventing post-operative recurrence of bladder cancer as BCG (Bacillus Calmette-Guérin) and greater than Mitomycin C (MMC)[32,33]. One study of 313 patients after TURBT (transurethral resection of bladder tumour) or partial cystectomy who were followed up for 2 to 15 years (average 7.6 years) reported recurrence rates of 34.9% in the group receiving *P. umbellatus* polysaccharide extract, compared with 35.1% in the BCG group, 41.7% in the MMC group and 64.7% in the control group[34].

In animal experiments *P. umbellatus* also inhibited the development of bladder cancer in rats exposed to N-butyl-N-(4-hydroxybutyl) nitrosamine with 11 of 18 animals staying cancer free. Polysaccharide extracts of *Lentinus edodes, Grifola frondosa* and *Pleurotus ostreatus* showed similar increases in host resistance with 9 of 17, 13 of 20 and 7 of 15 animals staying cancer free[35].

In vitro studies with *G. frondosa* and *Phellinus linteus* extracts showed synergistic action with vitamin C against bladder cancer cell lines with non-cytotoxic doses of polysaccharide extracts becoming highly cytotoxic in combination with non-toxic levels of vitamin C[36].

Brain Cancer Io Gf

Betulinic acid, a major component of aqueous extracts from *Inonotus obliquus* grown on birch trees, exerted cytotoxic activity against primary tumour cells cultured from patients in 4 of 4 medulloblastoma-tumour samples and in 20 of 24 glioblastoma-tumour samples with induction of apoptosis, while being non-toxic against mouse nerve cells[37-39].

Maitake D-fraction in combination with Maitake (*Grifola frondosa*) fruiting body was reported by Nanba to produce tumour regression or significant symptom improvement in 37% of brain cancer patients[40].

Breast Cancer Gf Tv

Polysaccharide extracts from *Lentinus edodes*, *Grifola frondosa* and *Trametes versicolor* have all been reported to be beneficial for breast cancer[41].

Long term immunotherapy with PSK has been shown to significantly improve the survival rate of patients with breast cancer[42], while a separate study in breast cancer patients with vascular invasion linked the effect of PSK supplementation to B40 antigen status (a known indicator of breast cancer survival) with 100% of B40-positive patients treated with PSK as well as chemotherapy surviving beyond 10 years, while for B40-negative patients the 10-year survival rate was approximately 50%[44].

Symptomatic improvement or regression was also reported by Nanba for 11 out of 15 breast cancer patients treated with a combination of Maitake D-fraction and Maitake (*G. frondosa*) fruiting body[40]. Mizuno reported recovery in a breast cancer patient with lung metastases using *Agaricus brasiliensis* polysaccharide extract[45], while *Phellinus linteus* has traditionally been used to treat breast cancer in Korea and polysaccharide extracts show strong *in vitro* activity[46].

Breast Cancer - Oestrogen independent Gl Pl

The transcription factor NF-kB has been identified as a key component in the ability of breast cancer cells to multiply independently of oestrogen while resisting chemotherapy and avoiding apoptosis[41].

Ganoderma lucidum has shown the most significant inhibitory effect on NF-kB in highly invasive breast cancer cells with the triterpenes particularly active. Triterpenes from *G. lucidum* have also been shown to inhibit aromatase activity, as well as the transcription factor AP1 (characteristic of highly metastatic breast cancer cells), while the clinical role of a triterpene-enriched *G. lucidum* extract in inhibiting NF-kB in a case of breast cancer is also reported in one paper[47].

In addition triterpenes from *Ganoderma lucidum* show Epstein-Barr virus inhibitory activity[41].

Other mushrooms which have demonstrated NF-kB inhibition *in vitro* include *Phellinus linteus* and *Lentinus edodes*.

Breast Cancer - Preventative Fv

There is growing evidence to suggest a protective effect against breast cancer from regular dietary intake of mushrooms, especially in post-menopausal women, and some evidence that the protective effect is enhanced in combination with green tea consumption.

An epidemiological study of 2,000 Chinese women, half with breast cancer and half without, found a reduction in risk of breast cancer in those women who regularly consumed mushrooms (10g/day fresh or 4g/day dried) and drank green tea (1.05g/day dried green tea leaves) with an increased reduction in women who did both[48]. A Korean study comparing 362 women with histologically confirmed breast cancer and an equal number of women without, matched by age and menopausal status, found a strong inverse correlation between mushroom consumption and breast cancer risk in postmenopausal women but not in pre-menopausal women[49]. *In vitro* studies with extracts of *Ganoderma lucidum* and green tea also showed synergistic effect in inhibiting adhesion, migration and invasion of oestrogen-independent and highly metastatic human breast cancer cells[50].

There is no data on which mushrooms were consumed in the above Chinese and Korean studies but in an *in vitro* study of aqueous extracts from 38 culinary and medicinal mushrooms, *Flammulina velutipes*, consumption of which has separately been linked to significant reductions in mortality, showed high levels of activity against both oestrogen +ve and -ve breast cancer cell lines, with almost complete inhibition (99%) of colony formation in oestrogen +ve cells and exceptionally rapid apoptosis of both oestrogen +ve and -ve cells[51]. In addition several culinary mushrooms, together with *G. lucidum* and multiple strains of *Fomitopsis officinalis*, demonstrate an ability to inhibit the enzyme aromatase, which converts androgen to oestrogen and whose abnormal expression in breast tissue is considered to be a risk factor for breast cancer[53]. Among the culinary mushrooms tested, which did not include *F. velutipes*, the common button mushroom, *Agaricus bisporus* had the highest anti-aromatase activity, followed by *Auricularia auricula*, *Pleurotus ostreatus* and *Lentinus edodes*.

Cervical Cancer Tv Ab

Schizophyllan (Sizofiran), a polysaccharide extract of *Schizophyllan commune*, is licensed in Japan for the treatment of cervical cancer and, in a 5-year multi-centre study, has been shown to significantly extend time to recurrence and improve survival rates in patients with stage II cervical cancer but not in those with stage III cancer[53,54]. A polysaccharide extract of *Agaricus brasiliensis* was shown to enhance NK cell activity in patients with gynaecological cancers (cervical, uterine and endometrial) undergoing chemotherapy (either carboplatin plus etoposide or carboplatin plus taxol) and reduce side effects from the chemotherapy (appetite suppression, alopecia, emotional stability and general weakness)[55].

Fve, a protein from *Flammulina velutipes*, significantly enhanced immune response to vaccination against HPV in an animal model and, in early stage cervical dysplasia (LSIL), *Trametes versicolor* biomass (3g/day) significantly increased the percentage of women showing normal cytology after 1 year (72.5% compared to 47.5% in the control group) and increased clearance of associated high risk HPV strains (91.5% vs. 8.5%)[56,57].

Colorectal Cancer Tv Gl Po Le

A recent meta-analysis of 3 clinical trials in Japan with 1,094 patients showed clear benefit from PSK supplementation (3.0g/day) in improving both survival and disease-free survival in cases of curatively resected colorectal cancer[58,59]. Chihara et al also report excellent results from a 4 year follow-up of Lentinan in phase III patients with colorectal cancer[60].

In a study on patients with advanced colorectal cancer, a polysaccharide extract from *Ganoderma lucidum* (5.4g/day) produced improvements in immune parameters with increases in mitogenic reactivity to phytohemagglutinin, counts of CD3, CD4, CD8 and CD56 lymphocytes, plasma concentrations of interleukin (IL)-2, IL-6 and interferon-gamma, and NK-cell activity, and decreases in plasma concentrations of IL-1 and tumour necrosis factor-alpha[61].

It is also likely that dietary consumption of mushrooms might be beneficial in reducing incidences of colon cancer due to their high content of dietary fibre and immune modulating activity, with *Pleurotus ostreatus* given at 5% of feed showing a protective effect on the development of dimethylhydrazine-induced colon cancer in rats[62,63]. Extracts from *G. lucidum* and *Lentinus edodes* also show protective effects against colon cancer development[64,65].

Endometrial Cancer   Ab

Agaricus brasiliensis polysaccharide extract enhanced NK cell activity in gynaecological cancer patients (including endometrial) undergoing chemotherapy (either carboplatin plus etoposide or carboplatin plus taxol) and reduced side effects from the chemotherapy[56].

Gastric Cancer (Stomach cancer)   Tv Le

Previously the most common cancer in Japan[66], mushroom polysaccharide extracts form part of mainstream treatment and their effects have been evaluated in several large scale clinical trials with very positive results.

A recent meta-analysis of trials with PSK including 8,009 patients confirmed improved survival of patients after curative gastric cancer resection and an individual patient data meta-analysis of 690 patients from 5 trials with Lentinan showed it to offer a significant advantage over chemotherapy alone in terms of survival for patients with advanced gastric cancer[67,68].

Leukaemia   Gf Ab

Clinical trials with PSK failed to show any statistically significant benefit[1] but Nanba et al reported reductions in CD4+ (-26%) and IL-2 (-17%) in 3 leukaemia cases with a combination of Maitake D-fraction and Maitake (*Grifola frondosa*) fruiting body[69].

In vitro experiments with polysaccharide extracts from several mushrooms, including *Agaricus brasiliensis, Ganoderma lucidum, Poria cocos, Trametes versicolor* and *Cordyceps sinensis* show activity against human leukaemia cell lines through induction of apoptosis, as do triterpenes from *G. lucidum* and *Antrodia camphorata*[70-80], while *in vivo* and *in vitro* studies with *A. brasiliensis* polysaccharide extracts showed tumour-selective growth inhibitory activity against human leukaemia cells[81].

Liver Cancer   Gf Gl Ac

Nanba et al reported that 7 of 12 patients with liver cancer responded to a combination of *Grifola frondosa* fruiting body (4-6g/day) and purified polysaccharide extract (MD fraction - 40-150mg/day)[40].

Studies using implanted sarcoma 180 as a model for liver cancer have shown inhibition of tumour rates of 52.8%, 56.6% and 51.9% when given polysaccharide extracts of *Flammulina velutipes*, *Lentinus edodes* and *Agaricus brasiliensis* respectively[82] and a 71.6% increase in lifespan of tumour-bearing mice with *Polyporus umbellatus* polysaccharide extract (i.p.) on its own and a 119.9% increase when given in conjunction with mitomycin C[83].

Several *in vitro* studies on *Ganoderma lucidum* and *G. lucidum* triterpenes have demonstrated cell growth inhibition and anti-invasive effects by multiple mechanisms including suppression of protein kinase C, activation of protein kinases, G2-phase cell cycle arrest, inactivation of MAPK/ERK signal transduction pathway and inhibition of the binding activities of NF-kB and AP-1[84-89]. In a human tumour xenograft model, a dose-response inhibition was also observed in the average size, volume, and weight of tumours upon oral administration of *G. lucidum* extract[90].

Antrodia camphorata has traditionally been used in the treatment of liver cancer in Taiwan. *In vitro* studies confirm its apoptotic effects on human liver cancer cell lines and a number of promising cases have been reported combining it with conventional treatment in cases of advanced liver cancer[91,92].

Cordyceps sinensis, *Pleurotus ostreatus* and *Inonotus obliquus* have all shown *in vitro* efficacy against liver cancer cell lines[93-95].

Lung Cancer Tv Gf

Trametes versicolor polysaccharide extracts show impressive benefits in cases of lung cancer.

In a 1993 study on patients with stage I-III non-small cell lung cancer treated with radiotherapy and PSK, PSK extended 5-yr survival 2-4x for all stages with maximum benefit in patients over the age of 70 and for tumours less than 5cm in diameter. In a 2003 study with non-small-cell lung cancer patients post-radiotherapy, those patients who received 3g PSK daily in 2 week cycles (2 weeks on, 2 weeks off) were almost 4 times more likely to be alive after 5 years than those without PSK (27% vs. 7%), with stage III patients who received PSK having a better prognosis than stage I/II patients who did not[96].

Grifola frondosa polysaccharide extract/fruiting body combination has also been reported to produce improvement in 65% of lung cancer patients[40].

Lymphoma Gl Tv

A number of papers report beneficial immunological effects of extracts from *Trametes versicolor* and *Ganoderma lucidum* in human lymphoma cell lines[97-101]. PSK was also reported to inhibit lymphoma development in a mouse model and a case of regression of gastric large B-Cell lymphoma following high *G. lucidum* intake has been reported[102,103].

Ovarian Cancer Tv Ab

PSK has been shown to reduce chemotherapy-induced IL2 suppression in ovarian cancer patients and to increase the survival rate of mice with human ovarian cancer[104-106]. PSK also showed combined benefit with cisplatin, a finding confirmed by *in vitro* studies[107].

A polysaccharide extract of *A. brasiliensis* was reported to increase NK cell activity and improve quality of life in patients with ovarian cancer, as well as other gynaecological cancers[56].

Pancreatic Cancer Tv

There have been two reports of unresectable pancreatic cancer responding to combined chemotherapy and PSK/Lentinan and one *in vitro* study showing PSK enhancing docetaxel induced apoptosis through NF-kB inhibition[108-110].

A compound has also been identified from *Antrodia camphorata* with toxicity against pancreatic cancer cells[71].

Prostate Cancer `Gl`

Ganoderma lucidum has been identified as a promising agent for prostate cancer with *in vitro* evidence showing inhibition of hormone dependent and independent prostate cancer cells through multiple pathways, including binding to androgen receptor, inhibition of the active transcription factors: NF-kB and AP-1, inhibition of urokinase-type plasminogen activator (uPA) and its receptor uPAR, as well as cell adhesion and cell migration of highly invasive breast and prostate cancer cells[111-122].

Ganodermic triterpenes have also been shown to suppress steroid 5α-reductase, which converts testosterone to dihydrotestosterone (DHT) and has been shown to play an important role in the development of prostate cancer and benign prostatic hyperplasia (BPH). The use of other steroid 5α-reductase inhibitors has been found to decrease the incidence of prostate cancer and *G. lucidum* would appear to be a promising candidate for further research in this regard.

Several *in vitro* studies using mushroom polysaccharides have also shown suppression of both androgen dependent and independent cell growth with a comparative study of aqueous extracts from 23 mushroom species, including *G. lucidum*, *Trametes versicolor*, *Grifola frondosa*, *Cordyceps sinensis*, *Agaricus brasiliensis*, *Lentinus edodes* and *Hericium erinaceus*, on androgen-independent PC-3 cells showing *Pleurotus ostreatus* and *Flammulina velutipes* to have the greatest cytotoxicity, significantly increasing cancer cell apoptosis[123,124]. *Coprinus comatus* has also been shown to reduce androgen and glucocorticoid receptor transcriptional activity in a dose dependent manner[125].

In addition, an *in vivo* study using severely immunodeficient mice found *A. brasiliensis* polysaccharides to directly inhibit the growth of prostate cancer cells via an apoptotic pathway and suppress prostate tumour growth via antiproliferative and antiangiogenic mechanisms[126].

However, a 2002 clinical study of a *L. edodes* polysaccharide extract showed it to be ineffective in stopping the disease with no instances of regression and progression in 23 of 61 men over a 6 month period[127].

Skin Cancer (Melanoma) `Gf` `Cs` `Tv`

In one *in vivo* study, injection of Maitake D-fraction produced 27% inhibition of a melanoma cell line in mice at a dose of 1mg/kg[128], while in others an ethanol extract of *Cordyceps sinensis* was effective at inhibiting growth of melanoma in the lungs of mice[129,130] and PSK at suppressing lung metastases of mouse melanoma[131].

Extracts of *Inonotus obliquus* and *Lentinus edodes* have also shown *in vitro* activity against melanoma cells lines[132,133], while triterpenes from *Poria cocos* have demonstrated anti-inflammatory activity and inhibition of the development of skin cancer in a mouse model[134,135].

CLINICAL NOTES

Oral dosage of polysaccharide/proteoglycan extracts such as PSK is typically 3-6g/day, although for long term supplementation this is sometimes reduced to every other day or given in weekly cycles (1 week on, 1 week off).

Dosages of dried herb material or biomass products can be considerably higher with doses of 15-50g/day reported for supplementation with mushroom biomass products in cancer cases and up to 300g/day for dried herb material.

As mushroom polysaccharide extracts not only strengthen immune response but also enhance the efficacy of conventional treatment, while at the same time reducing its side effects, it is beneficial to start supplementation as soon as cancer is diagnosed or suspected, continuing during any conventional treatment and for 3-6 months after. It can then be appropriate to continue with low dose supplementation to support immune health and help prevent recurrence, either daily or on alternate days or weeks (epidemiological studies show benefits from consuming mushrooms three or more times a week).

There is some in vitro evidence to suggest that co-administration of Vitamin C can increase effectiveness of mushroom polysaccharide supplementation in cancer therapy, with non-toxic doses of polysaccharide extracts from both Grifola frondosa (Maitake) and Phellinus linteus found to be strongly cytotoxic to bladder cancer cells when combined with a non-toxic dose of vitamin C, producing over 90% cell death[36]. Similar results were seen by Fullerton et. al. with G. frondosa polysaccharide extracts[136].

Transfer factors have also been suggested as beneficial adjuvants to mushroom nutrition supplementation[137].

For discussion on the use of medicinal mushrooms in cancer prevention see Breast Cancer - Prevention.

REFERENCES

1. The use of mushroom glucans and proteoglycans in cancer treatment. Kidd P.M. Altern Med Rev. 2000;5(1):4-27
2. Advances in immunomodulating studies of PSP. Li K.Y. Hong Kong Assoc. for Health Care Ltd. 1999;Advanced Research in PSP:39-46
3. A new biological response modifier - PSP. Yang Q.Y, Yi J.H, Li X.Y. 1993;PSP International Symposium:56-72
4. Polysaccharide peptide (PSP) restores immunosuppression induced by cyclophosphamide in rats. Qian Z.M, Xu M.F, Tang P.L. Am J Chin Med. 1997;25(1):27-35
5. Tsukagoshi S.Y, Hashimoto G, Fujii H, Kobayashi K, Nomoto, Orita K. Krestin (PSK). Cancer Treatment Review. 1984;11:131-155
6. Polysaccharopeptides derived from *Coriolus versicolor* potentiate the S-phase specific cytotoxicity of Camptothecin (CPT) on human leukaemia HL-60 cells. Wan J.M, Sit WH, Yang X, Jiang P, Wong L.L. Chin Med. 2010;5:16
7. Polysaccharopeptide enhances the anticancer activity of doxorubicin and etoposide on human breast cancer cells ZR-75-30. Wan J.M, Sit W.H, Louie J.C. Int J Oncol. 2008; 32(3):689-99
8. Enhancement of anti-cancer activity of cisdiaminedichloroplatinum by the protein-bound polysaccharide of *Coriolus versicolor* QUEL (PS-K) *in vitro*. Kobayashi Y, Kariya K, Saigenji K, Nakamura K. Cancer Biother. 1994;9(4):351-8

9. Antitumour effect of PSK and its combined effect with CDDP on ovarian serous adenocarcinoma-bearing nude mice. Ishii K, Kita T, Hirata J, Tode T, Kikuchi Y, Nagata I. Nippon Sanka Fujinka Gakkai Zasshi. 1993;45(4):333-9

10. Effects of PSK on interleukin-2 production by peripheral lymphocytes of patients with advanced ovarian carcinoma during chemotherapy. Kikuchi Y, Kizawa I, Oomori K, Iwano I, Kita T, Kato K. Jpn J Cancer Res. 1988;79(1):125-30

11. End-point result of a randomised controlled study on the treatment of gastrointestinal cancer with a combination of Lentinan and chemotherapeutic agents. Taguchi T, Furue H et.al. Excerpta Medica. 1985:151-165

12. Protective effect of *Armillaria mellea* polysaccharide on mice bone marrow cell damage caused by cyclophosphamide. Li Y.P, Wu K.F, Liu Y. Zhongguo Zhong Yao Za Zhi. 2005;30(4):283-6

13. *Hericium erinaceus* enhances doxorubicin-induced apoptosis in human hepatocellular carcinoma cells. Lee J.S, Hong E.K. Cancer Lett. 2010 May

14. Interaction of *Ganoderma* triterpenes with doxorubicin and proteomic characterization of the possible molecular targets of *Ganoderma triterpenes*. Yue Q.X, Xie F.B, Guan S.H, Ma C, Yang M, Jiang B.H, Liu X, Guo D.A. Cancer Sci. 2008;99(7):1461-70

15. Prevention of cisplatin induced nephrotoxicity by terpenes isolated from *Ganoderma lucidum* occurring in southern parts of India. Pillai TG, John M, Sara Thomas G. Exp Toxicol Pathol. 2009 Dec

16. Maitake beta-glucan enhances therapeutic effect and reduces myelo-supression and nephrotoxicity of cisplatin in mice. Masuda Y, Inoue M, Miyata A, Mizuno S, Nanba H. Int Immunopharmacol. 2009;9(5):620-6

17. *Cordyceps sinensis* health supplement enhances recovery from taxol-induced leukopenia. Liu W.C, Chuang W.L, Tsai M.L, Hong J.H, McBride W.H, Chiang C.S. Exp Biol Med (Maywood). 2008;233(4):447-55

18. Clinical evaluation of sizofran as assistant immunotherapy in treatment of head and neck cancer. Kimura Y et al. Acta Otolarynzology. 1994;511:192-195

19. Activated (HLA-DR+) T-lymphocyte subset in cervical carcinoma and effects of radiotherapy and immunotherapy with sizofiran on cell-mediated immunity and survival. Miyazaki K et al. Gynaecology and Oncology. 1995;56:412-420

20. Activation of peritoneal macrophages by polysaccharopeptide from the mushroom, *Coriolus versicolor*. Liu W.K, Ng T.B, Sze S.F, Tsui K.W. Immunopharmacology. 1993;26(2):139-46

21. Induction of apoptosis in human prostatic cancer cells with beta-glucan (Maitake mushroom polysaccharide). Fullerton S.A, Samadi A.A, Tortorelis D.G, Choudhury M.S, Mallouh C, Tazaki H, Konno S. Mol Urol. 2000;4(1):7-13

22. Pro- and antioxidative properties of medicinal mushroom extracts. Wei S, Griensven LJLD. Int J Med Mushr. 2008;10(4):30

23. Chemotherapy-induced thrombosis. Haddad T.C, Greeno E.W. Thromb Res. 2006;118(5):555-68

24. The effect of Tremella polysaccharides on leukopoenia following radiotherapy. Dai H. Chinese Pharmaceutical Journal 2006;41(13)p:1033-4

25. Radioprotective mechanism of preparation extracted from TFB. Effects on hemopoietic system in mice Xu C.X, Li Z.W, Yang F.T, Niu H.S, Liu S.H and Lu R.S Acta Academiae Medicinae Sinicae. 1984-05

26. Effect of *Tremella fuciformis* Berk on acute radiation sickness in dogs. Zhao T.F, Xu C.X, Li Z.W, Xie F, Zhao Y.T, Wang S.Q, Luo C.H and Lu R.S, Ni G.L , Ku Z.Q, Ni Y.F, Qian Q, Chen X.Q. Acta Academiae Medicinae Sinicae. 1982-01

27. The ameliorative effect of PSP on the toxic and side effect reactions of chemo- and radiotherapy of cancers. Advanced research in PSP. Sun Z et al. Hong Kong Association for Health Care Ltd. 1999:304-307

28. The use of Coriolus-MRL supplementation in lung cancer patients undergoing radiotherapy. Catita J. Mycology News. 2000;1(4):3-4

29. Protection against radiation-induced bone marrow and intestinal injuries by *Cordyceps sinensis*, a Chinese herbal medicine. Liu W.C, Wang S.C, Tsai M.L, Chen M.C, Wang Y.C, Hong J.H, McBride W.H, Chiang C.S. Radiat Res. 2006;166(6):900-7

30. A phase II multicenter, double-blind, randomized, placebo-controlled study of three dosages of an immunomodulator (PGG-glucan) in high-risk surgical patients. Babineau T.J, Hackford A, Kenler A, Bistrian B, Forse R.A, Fairchild P.G, Heard S, Keroack M, Caushaj P, Benotti P. Arch Surg. 1994;129(11):1204-10

31. Effect of PGG-glucan on the rate of serious postoperative infection or death observed after high-risk gastrointestinal operations. Betafectin Gastrointestinal Study Group. Dellinger E.P, Babineau T.J, Bleicher P, Kaiser A.B, Seibert G.B, Postier R.G, Vogel S.B, Norman J, Kaufman D, Galandiuk S, Condon R.E. Arch Surg. 1999;134(9):977-83

32. Inhibitory effect of Chinese herb medicine zhuling on urinary bladder cancer. An experimental and clinical study. Yang D.A. Zhonghua Wai Ke Za Zhi. 1991;29(6):393-5,399

33. Prophylactic effects of zhuling and BCG on postoperative recurrence of bladder cancer. Zhonghua Wai Ke Za Zhi. Yang D.A, Li S.Q, Li X.T. 1994;32(7):433-4

34. Prevention of postoperative recurrence of bladder cancer: a clinical study. Yang D, Li S, Wang H, Li X, Liu S, Han W, Hao J, Zhang H. Zhonghua Wai Ke Za Zhi. 1999;37(8):464-5

35. Effects of *Lentinus edodes*, *Grifola frondosa* and *Pleurotus ostreatus* administration on cancer outbreak, and activities of macrophages and lymphocytes in mice treated with a carcinogen, N-butyl-N-butanol-nitrosoamine. Kurashige S, Akuzawa Y, Endo F. Immunopharmacol Immunotoxicol. 1997;19(2):175-83

36. Effect of various natural products on growth of bladder cancer cells: two promising mushroom extracts. Konno S. Altern Med Rev. 2007;12(1):63-8

37. Betulinic acid: a new cytotoxic agent against malignant brain-tumour cells. Fulda S, Jeremias I, Steiner H.H, Pietsch T, Debatin K.M. Int J Cancer. 1999;82(3):435-41

38. Chemistry, biological activity, and chemotherapeutic potential of betulinic acid for the prevention and treatment of cancer and HIV infection. Cichewicz R.H, Kouzi S.A. Med Res Rev. 2004;24(1):90-114

39. Betulinic acid, a natural compound with potent anticancer effects. Mullauer F.B, Kessler J.H, Medema J.P. Anticancer Drugs. 2010;21(3):215-27

40. Maitake D-fraction: healing and preventive potential for cancer. Nanba H. J Orthomolecular Med. 1997;12:43-49

41. Potential Role of Medicinal Mushrooms in Breast Cancer Treatment: Current Knowledge and Future Perspectives. Petrova RD, Wasser SP; Mahajna JA, Denchev CM, Neva E. Intl J Med Mush. 2005;7(1-2):141-153

42. Hormone conditioned cancer chemotherapy for recurrent breast cancer prolongs survival. Sugimachi K, Inokuchi K, Matsuura H, Ueo H, Kumashiro R. Jpn J Surg. 1984 May;14(3):217-21

43. Immunochemotherapies versus chemotherapy as adjuvant treatment after curative resection of operable breast cancer. Iino Y, Yokoe T, Maemura M, Horiguchi J, Takei H, Ohwada S, Morishita Y. Anticancer Res. 1995 Nov-Dec;15(6B):2907-11

44. HLA antigen as predictive index for the outcome of breast cancer patients with adjuvant immunochemotherapy with PSK. Yokoe T, Iino Y, Takei H, Horiguchi J, Koibuchi Y, Maemura M, Ohwada S, Morishita Y. Anticancer Res. 1997 Jul-Aug;17(4A):2815-8

45. Medicinal properties and clinical effects of culinary-medicinal mushroom *Agaricus blazei* Murrill (Agaricomycetideae) (Review). Mizuno T. Int J Med Mushr. 2002;4:299–312

46. *Phellinus linteus* suppresses growth, angiogenesis and invasive behaviour of breast cancer cells through the inhibition of AKT signalling. Sliva D, Jedinak A, Kawasaki J, Harvey K, Slivova V. Br J Cancer. 2008;98(8): 1348-56

47. Potential Benefits of Ling Zhi or Reishi Mushroom *Ganoderma lucidum* (W. Curt.: Fr.) P. Karst. (Aphyllophoromycetideae) to Breast Cancer Patients. Chen A.W, Seleen J. Int J Med Mushr. 2007;9(1):29-38

48. Dietary intakes of mushrooms and green tea combine to reduce the risk of breast cancer in Chinese women. Zhang M, Huang J, Xie X, Holman C.D. Int J Cancer. 2009;124(6):1404-8

49. A case-control study on the dietary intake of mushrooms and breast cancer risk among Korean women. Hong S.A, Kim K, Nam S.J, Kong G, Kim M.K. Int J Cancer. 2008; 122(4):919–23

50. Combined effect of green tea and *Ganoderma lucidum* on invasive behavior of breast cancer cells. Thyagarajan A, Zhu J, Sliva D. Int J Oncol. 2007;30(4):963-9

51. in vitro effects on proliferation, apoptosis and colony inhibition in ER-dependent and ER-independent human breast cancer cells by selected mushroom species. Gu Y.H, Leonard J. Oncol Rep. 2006;15(2):417-23

52. Chemopreventive properties of mushrooms against breast cancer and prostate cancer. Chen S, Phung S, Kwok S, Ye J, Hur G, Oh S, Smith D, Yuan Y.C, Karlsberg K, Lui K. Int J Med Mush. 2005;3:342-343

53. Clinical evaluation of schizophyllan combined with irradiation in patients with cervical cancer. A randomized controlled study. Okamura K, Suzuki M, Chihara T, Fujiwara A, Fukuda T, Goto S, Ichinohe K, Jimi S, Kasamatsu T, Kawai N, et al. Cancer. 1986;58(4):865-72

54. Clinical evaluation of sizofiran combined with irradiation in patients with cervical cancer. A randomized controlled study; a five-year survival rate. Okamura K, Suzuki M, Chihara T, Fujiwara A, Fukuda T, Goto S, Ichinohe K, Jimi S, Kasamatsu T, Kawai N, et al. Biotherapy. 1989;1(2):103-7

55. Natural killer cell activity and quality of life were improved by consumption of a mushroom extract, *Agaricus blazei* Murill Kyowa, in gynecological cancer patients undergoing chemotherapy. Ahn W.S, Kim D.J, Chae D.J, Lee J.M, Bae S.M, Sin J.I, Kim Y.W, Namkoong S.E, Lee I.P. International Journal of Gynecological Cancer: 2004;14(4):589-594

56. Coadministration of the fungal immunomodulatory protein FIP-Fve and a tumour-associated antigen enhanced antitumour immunity. Ding Y, Seow S.V, Huang C.H, Liew L.M, Lim Y.C, Kuo I.C, Chua K.Y. Immunology. 2009;128(1 Sup):e881-94

57. *Coriolus versicolor* supplementation in HPV patients. Couto S, da Silva D.P. 20th European Congress of Obstetrics and Gynaecology, 2008

58. Efficacy of adjuvant immunochemotherapy with poly-saccharide K for patients with curatively resected colorectal cancer: a meta-analysis of centrally randomized controlled clinical trials. Sakamoto J, Morita S, Oba K, Matsui T, Kobayashi M, Nakazato H, Ohashi Y. Cancer Immunol Immunother. 2006;55(4):404-11

59. Monitoring of immune responses to a herbal immuno-modulator in patients with advanced colorectal cancer. Chen X, Hu Z.P, Yang X.X, Huang M, Gao Y, Tang W, Chan S.Y, Dai X, Ye J, Ho P.C, Duan W, Yang H.Y, Zhu Y.Z, Zhou S.F. Int Immunopharmacol. 2006;6(3):499-508

60. Antitumour and metastasis-inhibitory activities of lentinan as an immunomodulator: an overview. Chihara G, Hamuro J, Maeda Y.Y, Shiio T, Suga T, Takasuka N, Sasaki T. Cancer Detect Prev Suppl. 1987;1:423-43

61. Immune responses to water-soluble ling zhi mushroom *Ganoderma lucidum* (W.Curt.:Fr.) P. Karst. Polysaccharides in patients with advanced colorectal cancer. Huang M; Gao Y.H; Tang W; Dai X; Gao H; Chen G.L; Ye J.X; Chan E; Zhou S. Int J Med Mushr. 2006;7(4):525-538

62. Effect of oyster mushroom (*Pleurotus ostreatus*) on pathological changes in dimethylhydrazine-induced rat colon cancer. Bobek P, Galbavy S, Ozdin L. Oncol Rep. 1998;5(3):727-30

63. An aqueous polysaccharide extract from the edible mushroom *Pleurotus ostreatus* induces anti-proliferative and pro-apoptotic effects on HT-29 colon cancer cells. Lavi I, Friesem D, Geresh S, Hadar Y, Schwartz B. Cancer Lett. 2006;244(1):61-70

64. A water-soluble extract from cultured medium of *Ganoderma lucidum* (Rei-shi) mycelia suppresses azoxymethane-induction of colon cancers in male F344 rats. Lu H, Kyo E, Uesaka T, Katoh O, Watanabe H. Oncol Rep. 2003;10(2):375-9

65. Inhibition of human colon carcinoma development by lentinan from shiitake mushrooms (*Lentinus edodes*). Ng M.L, Yap A.T. J Altern Complement Med. 2002;8(5):581-9

66. Epidemiology of gastric cancer in Japan. Inoue M, Tsugane S. Postgrad Med J. 2005;81:419-424

67. Efficacy of adjuvant immunochemotherapy with polysaccharide K for patients with curative resections of gastric cancer. Oba K, Teramukai S, Kobayashi M, Matsui T, Kodera Y, Sakamoto J. Cancer Immunol Immunother. 2007;56(6):905-11

68. Individual patient based meta-analysis of lentinan for unresectable/ recurrent gastric cancer. Oba K, Kobayashi M, Matsui T, Kodera Y, Sakamoto J. Anticancer Res. 2009;29(7):2739-45

69. Can Maitake MD-fraction aid cancer patients? Kodama N, Komuta K, Nanba H. Alt Med Rev. 2002;7(3):236

70. *Ganoderma lucidum* causes apoptosis in leukaemia, lymphoma and multiple myeloma cells. Müller C.I, Kumagai T, O'Kelly J, Seeram N.P, Heber D, Koeffler H.P. Leuk Res. 2006;30(7):841-8

71. *Ganoderma lucidum* polysaccharides can induce human monocytic leukaemia cells into dendritic cells with immuno-stimulatory function. Chan W.K, Cheung C.C, Law H.K, Lau Y.L, Chan G.C. J Hematol Oncol. 2008;1:9

72. Antiproliferative and differentiating effects of polysaccharide fraction from fu-ling (*Poria cocos*) on human leukemic U937 and HL-60 cells. Chen Y.Y, Chang H.M. Food Chem Toxicol. 2004;42(5):759-69

73. *Coriolus versicolor* (Yunzhi) extract attenuates growth of human leukaemia xenografts and induces apoptosis through the mitochondrial pathway. Ho C.Y, Kim C.F, Leung K.N, Fung K.P, Tse T.F, Chan H, Lau C.B. Oncol Rep. 2006;16(3):609-16

74. Cytotoxic activities of *Coriolus versicolor* (Yunzhi) extract on human leukaemia and lymphoma cells by induction of apoptosis. Lau C.B, Ho C.Y, Kim C.F, Leung K.N, Fung K.P, Tse T.F, Chan H.H, Chow M.S. Life Sci. 2004;75(7):797-808

75. Primary mechanism of apoptosis induction in a leukaemia cell line by fraction FA-2-b-ss prepared from the mushroom *Agaricus blazei* Murill. Gao L, Sun Y, Chen C, Xi Y, Wang J, Wang Z. Braz J Med Biol Res. 2007;40(11):1545-55

76. *Cordyceps sinensis* mycelium extract induces human premyelocytic leukaemia cell apoptosis through mitochondrion pathway. Zhang Q.X, Wu J.Y. Exp Biol Med (Maywood). 2007;232(1):52-7

77. Effect of *Cordyceps sinensis* on the proliferation and differentiation of human leukemic U937 cells. Chen Y.J, Shiao M.S, Lee S.S, Wang S.Y. Life Sci. 1997;60(25):2349-59

78. *Ganoderma lucidum* causes apoptosis in leukaemia, lymphoma and multiple myeloma cells. Müller C.I, Kumagai T, O'Kelly J, Seeram N.P, Heber D, Koeffler H.P. Leuk Res. 2006;30(7):841-8

79. Lucidenic acid B induces apoptosis in human leukaemia cells via a mitochondria-mediated pathway. Hsu C.L, Yu Y.S, Yen G.C. J Agric Food Chem. 2008;56(11):3973-80

80. Compound MMH01 possesses toxicity against human leukaemia and pancreatic cancer cells. Chen Y.J, Chou C.J, Chang T.T. Toxicol in vitro. 2009;23(3):418-24
81. Inhibitory effects of *Agaricus blazei* extracts on human myeloid leukaemia cells. Kim C.F, Jiang J.J, Leung K.N, Fung K.P, Lau C.B. J Ethnopharmacol. 2009;122(2):320-6
82. Inhibitory activity of polysaccharide extracts from three kinds of edible fungi on proliferation of human hepatoma SMMC-7721 cell and mouse implanted S180 tumour. Jiang S.M, Xiao Z.M, Xu Z.H. World J Gastroenterol. 1999;5(5):404-407
83. Combined effects of chuling (*Polyporus umbellatus*) extract and mitomycin C on experimental liver cancer. You J.S, Hau D.M, Chen K.T, Huang H.F. Am J Chin Med. 1994;22(1):19-28
84. Triterpene-enriched extracts from *Ganoderma lucidum* inhibit growth of hepatoma cells via suppressing protein kinase C, activating mitogen-activated protein kinases and G2-phase cell cycle arrest. Lin S.B, Li C.H, Lee S.S, Kan LS. Life Sci. 2003;72(21):2381-90
85. Ganoderic acid produced from submerged culture of *Ganoderma lucidum* induces cell cycle arrest and cytotoxicity in human hepatoma cell line BEL7402. Yang H.L. Biotechnol Lett. 2005;27(12):835-8
86. Antitumour activity of the sporoderm-broken germinating spores of *Ganoderma lucidum*. Liu X, Yuan J.P, Chung C.K, Chen X.J. Cancer Lett. 2002;182(2):155-61
87. Ganoderiol F, a ganoderma triterpene, induces senescence in hepatoma HepG2 cells. Chang U.M, Li C.H, Lin L.I, Huang C.P, Kan L.S, Lin S.B. Life Sci. 2006;79(12):1129-39
88. The anti-invasive effect of lucidenic acids isolated from a new *Ganoderma lucidum* strain. Weng C.J, Chau C.F, Chen K.D, Chen D.H, Yen G.C. Mol Nutr Food Res. 2007;51(12):1472-7
89. Lucidenic acid inhibits PMA-induced invasion of human hepatoma cells through inactivating MAPK/ERK signal transduction pathway and reducing binding activities of NF-kappaB and AP-1. Weng C.J, Chau C.F, Hsieh Y.S, Yang S.F, Yen G.C. Carcinogenesis. 2008;29(1): 147-56
90. Inhibitory effects of *Ganoderma lucidum* on tumourigenesis and metastasis of human hepatoma cells in cells and animal models. Weng C.J, Chau C.F, Yen G.C, Liao J.W, Chen D.H, Chen K.D. J Agric Food Chem. 2009;57(11):5049-57
91. Apoptotic effects of extract from *Antrodia camphorata* fruiting bodies in human hepatocellular carcinoma cell lines. Hsu Y.L, Kuo Y.C, Kuo P.L, Ng L.T, Kuo Y.H, Lin C.C. Cancer Lett. 2005;221(1):77-89
92. Niuchangchih (*Antrodia camphorata*) and its potential in treating liver diseases. Ao Z.H, Xu Z.H, Lu Z.M, Xu HY, Zhang X.M, Dou W.F. J Ethnopharmacol. 2009;121(2):194-212
93. *Cordyceps sinensis* increases the expression of major histocompatibility complex class II antigens on human hepatoma cell line HA22T/VGH cells. Chiu J.H, Ju C.H, Wu L.H, Lui W.Y, Wu C.W, Shiao M.S, Hong C.Y. Am J Chin Med. 1998;26(2):159-70
94. A new lectin with highly potent antihepatoma and antisarcoma activities from the oyster mushroom *Pleurotus ostreatus*. Wang H, Gao J, Ng T.B. Biochem Biophys Res Commun. 2000;275(3):810-6
95. Chaga mushroom (*Inonotus obliquus*) induces G0/G1 arrest and apoptosis in human hepatoma HepG2 cells. Youn M.J, Kim J.K, Park S.Y, Kim Y, Kim S.J, Lee J.S, Chai K.Y, Kim H.J, Cui M.X, So H.S, Kim K.Y, Park R. World J Gastroenterol. 2008;14(4):511-7
96. *Coriolus versicolor* polysaccharide peptide slows progression of advanced non-small cell lung cancer. Tsang K.W, Lam C.L, Yan C, Mak J.C, Ooi G.C, Ho J.C, Lam B, Man R, Sham J.S, Lam W.K. Respir Med. 2003;97(6):618-24
97. Protein-bound polysaccharide-K (PSK) directly enhanced IgM production in the human B cell line BALL-1. Maruyama S, Akasaka T, Yamada K, Tachibana H. Biomed Pharmacother. 2009;63(6):409-12
98. Protein-bound polysaccharide K induced apoptosis of the human Burkitt lymphoma cell line, Namalwa. Hattori T.S, Komatsu N, Shichijo S, Itoh K.Biomed Pharmacother. 2004;58(4):226-30
99. *Ganoderma lucidum* causes apoptosis in leukaemia, lymphoma and multiple myeloma cells. Müller C.I, Kumagai T, O'Kelly J, Seeram N.P, Heber D, Koeffler H.P. Leuk Res. 2006;30(7):841-8
100. Cytotoxic action of *Ganoderma lucidum* on interleukin-3 dependent lymphoma DA-1 cells: involvement of apoptosis proteins. Calviño E, Pajuelo L, de Eribe Casas J.A, Manjón J.L, Tejedor M.C, Herráez A, Alonso M.D, Diez J.C. Phytother Res 2010 Jun
101. Potentiation of T cell immunity against radiation-leukaemia-virus-induced lymphoma by polysaccharide K. Yefenof E, Einat E, Klein E. Cancer Immunol Immunother. 1991;34(2):133-7
102. Prophylactic intervention in radiation-leukaemia-virus-induced murine lymphoma by the biological response modifier polysaccharide K. Yefenof E, Gafanovitch I, Oron E, Bar M, Klein E. Cancer Immunol Immunother. 1995;41(6):389-96
103. Regression of gastric large B-Cell lymphoma accompanied by a florid lymphoma-like T-cell reaction: immunomodulatory effect of *Ganoderma lucidum* (Lingzhi)? Cheuk W, Chan J.X, Nuovo G, Chan M.K, Fok M. Int J Surg Pathol. 2007;15(2):180-6
104. Effects of cimetidine and PSK on interleukin-2 production by PBL in patients with advanced ovarian carcinoma during the course of chemo-therapy. Kikuchi Y, Kizawa I, Oomori K, Iwano I, Kita T, Miyauchi M, Kato K. Nippon Sanka Fujinka Gakkai Zasshi. 1987;39(11):1987-92
105. Effects of PSK on interleukin-2 production by peripheral lymphocytes of patients with advanced ovarian carcinoma during chemotherapy. Kikuchi Y, Kizawa I, Oomori K, Iwano I, Kita T, Kato K. Jpn J Cancer Res. 1988;79(1):125-30
106. Antitumour effect of PSK and its combined effect with CDDP on ovarian serous adenocarcinoma-bearing nude mice. Ishii K, Kita T, Hirata J, Tode T, Kikuchi Y, Nagata I. Nippon Sanka Fujinka Gakkai Zasshi. 1993;45(4):333-9
107. Enhancement of anti-cancer activity of cisdiaminedichloroplatinum by the protein-bound polysaccharide of *Coriolus versicolor* QUEL (PS-K) in vitro. Kobayashi Y, Kariya K, Saigenji K, Nakamura K. Cancer Biother. 1994;9(4):351-8
108. Two cases of unresectable pancreatic cancer responding to combined chemotherapy with cisplatin, PSK and UFT. Sohma M, Kitagawa T, Okano S, Utsumi M, Mutoh E, Takeda S, Kanda M, Suzuki Y, Okamura K, Namiki M. Gan To Kagaku Ryoho. 1987;14(6 Pt 1):1926-9
109. A case of unresectable pancreatic cancer that responded to UFT chemotherapy. Gan No Rinsho. Sato Y, Sakai T, Okada T, Sasano Y, Ando T, Haruta J, Kanayama K, Kuwahara Y, Tachino H, Tahara H, et al. 1990;36(11):2073-8
110. PSK-mediated NF-kappaB inhibition augments docetaxel-induced apoptosis in human pancreatic cancer cells NOR-P1. Zhang H, Morisaki T, Nakahara C, Matsunaga H, Sato N, Nagumo F, Tadano J, Katano M. Oncogene. 2003;22(14):2088-96
111. Pharmacological values of medicinal mushrooms for prostate cancer therapy: the case of *Ganoderma lucidum*. Mahajna J, Dotan N, Zaidman B.Z, Petrova R.D, Wasser S.P. Nutr Cancer. 2009;61(1):16-26
112. *Ganoderma lucidum* (Reishi) in cancer treatment. Sliva D. Integr Cancer Ther. 2003;2(4):358-64. Androgen receptor-dependent and -independent mechanisms mediate Ganoderma lucidum activities in LNCaP prostate cancer cells. Zaidman B.Z, Wasser S.P, Nevo E, Mahajna J. Int J Oncol. 2007;31(4):959-67
113. Anti-androgen effects of extracts and compounds from *Ganoderma lucidum*. Liu J, Tamura S, Kurashiki K, Shimizu K, Noda K, Konishi F, Kumamoto S, Kondo R. Chem Biodivers. 2009;6(2):231-43
114. The anti-androgen effect of ganoderol B isolated from the fruiting body of *Ganoderma lucidum*. Liu J, Shimizu K, Konishi F, Kumamoto S, Kondo R. Bioorg Med Chem. 2007;15(14):4966-72

115. Medicinal mushroom cuts off prostate cancer cells' blood supply. Johnston N. Drug Discov Today. 2005;10(23-24):1584
116. *Ganoderma lucidum* suppresses angiogenesis through the inhibition of secretion of VEGF and TGF-beta1 from prostate cancer cells. Stanley G, Harvey K, Slivova V, Jiang J, Sliva D. Biochem Biophys Res Commun. 2005;330(1):46-52
117. *Ganoderma lucidum* inhibits proliferation and induces apoptosis in human prostate cancer cells PC-3. Jiang J, Slivova V, Valachovicova T, Harvey K, Sliva D. Int J Oncol. 2004;24(5):1093-9
118. Biologic activity of spores and dried powder from *Ganoderma lucidum* for the inhibition of highly invasive human breast and prostate cancer cells. Sliva D, Sedlak M, Slivova V, Valachovicova T, Lloyd F.P Jr, Ho N.W. J Altern Complement Med. 2003;9(4):491-7
119. Ganoderic acid DM: anti-androgenic osteoclastogenesis inhibitor. Liu J, Shiono J, Shimizu K, Kukita A, Kukita T, Kondo R. Bioorg Med Chem Lett. 2009;19(8):2154-7
120. Anti-androgenic activities of *Ganoderma lucidum*. Fujita R, Liu J, Shimizu K, Konishi F, Noda K, Kumamoto S, Ueda C, Tajiri H, Kaneko S, Suimi Y, Kondo R. J Ethnopharmacol. 2005;102(1):107-12
121. Androgen receptor-dependent and -independent mechanisms mediate *Ganoderma lucidum* activities in LNCaP prostate cancer cells. Zaidman B.Z, Wasser S.P, Nevo E, Mahajna J.Int J Oncol. 2007;31(4):959-67
122. Mushroom substances as therapeutics for hormone refractory prostate cancer. Mahajna J.A et al. Int J Med Mushr. 2007;9(3):212
123. Induction of apoptosis in human prostatic cancer cells with beta-glucan (Maitake mushroom polysaccharide). Fullerton S.A, Samadi A.A, Tortorelis D.G, Choudhury M.S, Mallouh C, Tazaki H, Konno S. Mol Urol. 2000;4(1):7-13
124. Cytotoxic effect of oyster mushroom *Pleurotus ostreatus* on human androgen-independent prostate cancer PC-3 cells. Gu Y.H, Sivam G. J Med Food. 2006;9(2):196-204
125. *Coprinus comatus* and *Ganoderma lucidum* interfere with androgen receptor function in LNCaP prostate cancer cells. Zaidman B.Z, Wasser S.P, Nevo E, Mahajna J. Mol Biol Rep. 2008;35(2):107-17
126. Inhibitory mechanisms of *Agaricus blazei* Murill on the growth of prostate cancer *in vitro* and *in vivo*. Yu C.H, Kan S.F, Shu C.H, Lu T.J, Sun-Hwang L, Wang P.S. J Nutr Biochem. 2009;20(10):753-64
127. Effects of a mushroom mycelium extract on the treatment of prostate cancer. deVere White R.W, Hackman R.M, Soares S.E, Beckett L.A, Sun B. Urology. 2002;60(4):640-4
128. Maitake D-fraction. Apoptosis inducer and immune enhancer. Konno S. Comp and Alt Ther. 2001;Apr:102-107
129. Effects of *Cordyceps sinensis* on natural killer activity and colony formation of B16 melanoma. Xu R.H, Peng X.E, Chen G.Z, Chen G.L.Chin Med J (Engl). 1992;105(2):97-101
130. Inhibitory effects of ethyl acetate extract of *Cordyceps sinensis* mycelium on various cancer cells in culture and B16 melanoma in C57BL/6 mice. Wu J.Y, Zhang Q.X, Leung P.H. Phytomedicine. 2007;14(1):43-9
131. Antimetastatic effect of PSK, a protein-bound polysaccharide, against the B16-BL6 mouse melanoma. Matsunaga K, Ohhara M, Oguchi Y, Iijima H, Kobayashi H. Invasion Metastasis. 1996;16(1):27-38
132. Selective induction of apoptosis in murine skin carcinoma cells (CH72) by an ethanol extract of *Lentinula edodes*. Gu Y.H, Belury M.A. Cancer Lett. 2005;220(1):21-8
133. Potential anticancer properties of the water extract of *Inonotus obliquus* by induction of apoptosis in melanoma B16-F10 cells. Youn M.J, Kim J.K, Park S.Y, Kim Y, Park C, Kim E.S, Park K.I, So H.S, Park R. J Ethnopharmacol. 2009;121(2):221-8
134. Inhibitory effects of lanostane-type triterpene acids, the components of *Poria cocos*, on tumour promotion by 12-O-tetradecanoylphorbol-13-acetate in two-stage carcinogenesis in mouse skin. Kaminaga T, Yasukawa K, Kanno H, Tai T, Nunoura Y, Takido M. Oncology. 1996;53(5):382-5
135. Triterpene acids from *Poria cocos* and their anti-tumour-promoting effects. Akihisa T, Nakamura Y, Tokuda H, Uchiyama E, Suzuki T, Kimura Y, Uchikura K, Nishino H. J Nat Prod. 2007;70(6):948-53
136. Induction of apoptosis in human prostatic cancer cells with beta-glucan (Maitake mushroom polysaccharide). Fullerton SA, Samadi AA, Tortorelis DG, Choudhury MS, Mallouh C, Tazaki H, Konno S. Mol Urol. 2000 Spring;4(1):7-13
137. Increased tumour necrosis factor alpha (TNF-alpha) and natural killer cell (NK) function using an integrative approach in late stage cancers. See D, Mason S, Roshan R. Immunol Invest. 2002;31(2):137-53

Medicinal Mushrooms for other conditions

Allergic Rhinitis (Hayfever) `Gl`

Ganoderma lucidum shows excellent results in the management of allergic rhinitis, its polysaccharides suppressing the pro-inflammatory, Th2 mediated immune state responsible for the hypersensitivity to the particular allergen(s) while several of its triterpenoid ganoderic and lucidenic acids have direct anti-inflammatory and anti-histamine action[1-4]. It thus addresses both the symptoms and the underlying imbalance of the condition and can be used in either a prophylactic or therapeutic mode.

> **CLINICAL NOTE**
>
> *Biomass is often effective in mild cases while triterpene-rich extracts have stronger anti-histamine activity for more severe cases - 1-3g/day.*

Alzheimers Disease (AD) `He` `Gl`

Low levels of nerve growth factor (NGF) are seen in AD with implications for the application of *Hericium erinaceus* in the management of this condition (see discussion on Dementia). In addition, synaptic degeneration, with loss of synaptic density proteins, has been shown to be a key mode of neurodegeneration in AD with beta-amyloid (Abeta) identified as a cause of synaptic dysfunction and contributor to AD pathology. *Ganoderma lucidum* aqueous extract, which has traditionally been considered to have anti-aging properties, has been shown to significantly inhibit Abeta-induced synaptotoxicity and also inhibit Abeta-triggered DEVD cleavage in a dose dependent manner with potential clinical application in management of AD[5].

> **CLINICAL NOTE**
>
> *H. erinaceus fruiting body and G. lucidum extract can be combined in the treatment of AD. 3g/day H. erinaceus fruiting body with 1g/day G. lucidum extract.*

Arrythmia `Cs`

Cordyceps sinensis has been reported as being used in the treatment of arrythmia in China and it has been suggested that this is at least partially due to the presence of adenosine, which is considered a class V antiarrhythmic agent[6].

> **CLINICAL NOTE**
>
> *Biomass products containing high levels of nucleoside derivatives - 3-6g/day.*

Asthma Cs Gl

Cordyceps sinensis has traditionally been used to treat respiratory disorders including asthma and serum markers of airway inflammation were seen to be reduced in patients with mild asthma given *C. sinensis* capsules[7]. *C. sinensis* also improved lung function in sensitized guinea pigs and reduced airway inflammation in sensitized rats[8]. An *in vitro* study on human airway epithelial cells showed *C. sinensis* and its components to alter ion transport and regulate Th1/Th2 balance[9,10].

Ganoderma lucidum has also traditionally been used to treat asthma and its triterpenoid components are known to have strong anti-inflammatory and anti-histamine activity. Research on a closely related species, *Ganoderma tsugae*, in murine models of allergic asthma shows that triterpenoid extracts reduce bronchoalveolar inflammation and attenuate Th2 responses without overall immunosuppressive effects[11,12].

In addition, mushroom polysaccharide extracts are known to shift immune balance away from Th2 dominance and towards Th1 dominance and have been shown to help correct a skewed Th1/Th2 balance in an animal asthma model, indicating their potential in the management of this condition, as well as other allergic disorders[13].

> **CLINICAL NOTE**
>
> *C. sinensis biomass combines well with triterpene-rich or triterpene/polysaccharide extracts from G. lucidum to treat a wide range of lung disorders. 3g/day C. sinensis biomass with 1-3g/day G. lucidum extract.*

Bacterial Infections He

Through their ability to strengthen the host immune response, fungal polysaccharides increase resistance and reduce incidences of post-surgical infection[14]. In addition, mushrooms have evolved a range of defences against other competing micro-organisms and several show direct anti-microbial action.

When aqueous extracts of *Lentinus edodes* and *Pleurotus ostreatus* were tested against a panel of 29 bacterial and 10 fungal pathogens, *L. edodes* extract showed extensive antimicrobial activity against 85% of the organisms, including 50% of the yeast and mould species, while aqueous extracts of *P. ostreatus* showed 87.5%

inhibition against E. coli and 57.5% against B. subtilis[15]. In a study of over 200 species of mushroom in Spain almost 50% had direct antibiotic activity against a range of test organisms[16].

Extracts of both *Hericium erinaceus* fruiting body and mycelium exhibited anti-MRSA activity with erinacines identified as active compounds. In clinical tests in Japan MRSA was seen to disappear in a number of patients given *H. erinaceus*[17]. Similar cyathane type compounds from other mushroom species also show antibiotic potential[18], while the traditional use of *H. erinaceus* in the treatment of gastritis (now known to be caused in many cases by the bacteria *H. pylori*) also indicates antibiotic properties.

CLINICAL NOTE
Traditionally H. erinaceus fruiting body has been used but the fact that the cyathane derivatives it contains have antibiotic properties points to probable excretion into the substrate with clinical possibilities for the biomass. Dosage of fruiting body prescribed in the Chinese Pharmacopoeia is 25-50g/day.

Benign Prostatic Hyperplasia (BPH) [Gf]

Triterpenoid compounds from *Ganoderma lucidum* have a marked anti-androgen effect, inhibiting 5alpha-reductase and significantly reducing testosterone-induced growth of the ventral prostate in rats[19-22].

Crude extracts from *Grifola frondosa* have also been reported to inhibit androgen-stimulated cell division in prostatic tissue *in vivo* at a dose of 500mg/kg. Purification of the polysaccharides did not result in greater levels of inhibition, suggesting that the active component is not polysaccharide-based or only partially polysaccharide-based.

CLINICAL NOTE
G. lucidum triterpene-rich extract - 1-3g/day.

Candidiasis [Tv] [Le]

Mushrooms are seen to exhibit both direct and indirect anti-fungal activity *in vitro* and *in vivo*[23]. The widely held belief that mushrooms somehow exacerbate candidal overgrowth runs contrary to scientific research, clinical experience and theoretical understanding. Not only do mushrooms stimulate the body's anti-fungal immune response but in nature they need to compete for resources with other fungi, as well as other microorganisms, and so have evolved a range of anti-fungal defences.

Lentinus edodes extracts and juice show strong anti-fungal action, as do aqueous extracts of *Pleurotus ostreatus,* with 50% inhibition against C. albicans[24-8]. In addition, triterpenes from Ganoderma species show anti-fungal activity[23], while mice given a polysaccharide-rich extract of *A. brasiliensis* showed enhanced candidacidal activity characterized by higher levels of H_2O_2 and increased mannose receptor expression by peritoneal macrophages (involved in the attachment and phagocytosis of non-opsonized microorganisms)[29].

It has also been suggested that chitin present in mushroom cell walls may help prevent colonisation of the intestinal mucosa by candida species[30].

Trametes versicolor has traditionally been used in Mexico to treat thrush and clinically is seen to reduce candidal overgrowth. PSK has also been shown to have a pronounced protective effect against lethal infection with *C. albicans* in mice. An injection of 250mg/kg 24 hours before inoculation of 1×10^6 *C. albicans* increased the 30 day survival rate by 60% and mean survival time by 209%[31]. Oral supplementation of tumour-bearing mice challenged with *C. albicans* was also increased by oral administration of PSK, together with a significant reduction in fungal counts[32].

CLINICAL NOTE

While polysaccharides are responsible for potentiating the immune response, many anti-fungal compounds produced by mushrooms are excreted into the substrate and captured by solid state fermentation (biomass).

T. versicolor and L. edodes biomass products show good anti-candida activity. 2-3g/day.

Chronic Fatigue Syndrome (CFS - ME)   [Tv] [Ps]

CFS patients show immune dysfunction, including low NK cell activity, and the condition has been linked to high viral counts, especially Epstein-barr virus (EBV). Recent research confirms the elevated levels of Th2 cytokines in patients with CFS and prevailing Th2 inflammatory milieu, together with highly attenuated Th1 immune response[33-35].

The proven ability of mushroom nutrition to promote a shift away from a Th2 dominant immune response and increase anti-viral activity makes it a natural source of support for CFS patients with good clinical results, including increased NK cell activity and improved lifestyle scores. *Trametes versicolor* biomass produced a 35% increase in NK cell activity in patients with mild CFS at a dose of 1.5-3g/day (more severe cases are reported to respond to higher dosages)[36].

CLINICAL NOTE

CFS is a condition that responds well to a range of medicinal mushrooms with polysaccharide extracts giving particularly good results. 1-3g/day.

Dementia He

Compounds in *Hericium erinaceus* are able to stimulate the production of nerve growth factor (NGF), which promotes repair and regeneration of neurons, and there is growing clinical evidence showing benefit for *H. erinaceus* in cases of mild dementia.

In a double-blind placebo controlled trial, 50-80-year old Japanese men and women with mild cognitive impairment given 3g/day *H. erinaceus* as tablets showed significant increases on a cognitive function scale compared with a placebo group over a 16 week period[37].

In another study 7 patients with different types of dementia were given 5g a day of *H. erinaceus* in soup. After six months all seven demonstrated improvement in their Functional Independence Measure score (eating, dressing, walking, etc.), while six out of seven demonstrated improvements in their perceptual capacities (understanding, communication, memory, etc.)[38].

> **CLINICAL NOTE**
>
> *The above clinical trials both used H. erinaceus fruiting body. 3-5g/day.*

Diabetes Cs

Fungal beta-glucans, along with beta-glucans from oats and barley, have been shown to help control blood glucose levels and it has been suggested that a possible mechanism is activation of P13K/Akt through binding to receptors including Dectin 1 and Scavenger[39]. However, daily supplementation of a normal diet with 3.5g/day beta-glucan in type II diabetics over 8 weeks failed to produce any change in fasting glucose levels[40].

Almost all of the common medicinal mushrooms have been investigated for benefit in different diabetes models, with results such as those given below:

Agaricus brasiliensis - Consumption of 1.5g of polysaccharide extract in combination with metformin and gliclazide for 12 weeks reduced insulin resistance in patients with type II diabetes[41].

Auricularia auricula - A water-soluble polysaccharide from *A. auricularia* at 3% of feed reduced fasting glucose levels and improved glucose tolerance in mice[42].

Cordyceps sinensis - Animal studies at a dose of 250mg/kg showed improved insulin sensitivity and reduced fasting blood glucose. In one clinical trial 3g/day of a proprietary *C. sinensis* preparation improved blood sugar control in 95% of patients compared to 54% of a control group treated by other methods[43-45].

Ganoderma lucidum - Consumption of 5.4g of polysaccharide extract for 8 weeks produced a 13% reduction in blood sugar levels in patients with type II diabetes mellitus who were not taking insulin and also led to significant improvement in peripheral neuropathy in diabetic patients[46,47].

Grifola frondosa - Improved glucose tolerance in diabetic rats at 20% of feed and in a separate experiment at 1g/day. A water soluble extract, X-fraction increases insulin sensitivity[48-50].

Hericium erinaceus - Blood sugar levels decreased by 19-26% in rats fed *H. erinaceus* extract at 100mg/kg[51].

Pleurotus ostreatus - Reduced plasma glucose levels at 4% of feed and was reported to reduce blood glucose in diabetic patients at an unspecified dosage[52,53].

Tremella fuciformis - 200mg/kg of a polysaccharide extract produced a 52% reduction in plasma glucose levels[54].

Some practitioners report good results with *Coprinus comatus* but published research either relates to vanadium-enriched *C. comatus* or to high supplementation levels[55-59].

CLINICAL NOTE

C. sinensis biomass at a dose of 3-5g/day can be helpful for stabilising blood sugar levels in both insulin dependent and non-insulin dependent diabetes and in reducing diabetes related depression.

Erectile Dysfunction Cs

Cordyceps sinensis has traditionally been used to treat male sexual dysfunction and *in vitro* and *in vivo* studies have shown it to increase the level of male hormones[61-63]. Clinical experience with *C. sinensis* biomass confirms its benefits in this area when taken over an extended period.

CLINICAL NOTE

3g/day biomass.

Fluid Retention Pu Pc

Polyporus umbellatus and *Poria cocos* are traditionally used in the treatment of fluid retention with *P. umbellatus* considered stronger. Multiple diuretic components have been isolated from *P. umbellatus*[64,65].

CLINICAL NOTE

Traditional dose is 6-15g dried herb.

Gastritis [He]

Hericium erinaceus has traditionally been used in the treatment of gastritis and extracts have been shown to be effective clinically and in animal models with reported inhibition rates of 70-90%[66,67,68].

> **CLINICAL NOTE**
>
> *Animal experiments showed maximum efficacy at a dose of 500mg/kg and the Chinese Pharmacopoeia gives a daily dose of 25-50g.*

Hepatitis [Cs] [Pu] [Gl] [Ps]

Several polysaccharide extracts have shown benefit in treatment of hepatitis B virus (HBV). Concentrated polysaccharide extracts from *Polyporus umbellatus* (92% polysaccharide) are used in China to treat patients with chronic HBV (40mg/day) with significant effect on clearing serum hepatitis B surface antigen (HBsAg) and HBV DNA[69,70], while a small study with *A. brasiliensis* polysaccharide extract (1500mg/day) in patients with HBV reported reductions in AST from 246 to 61.3 and ALT from 151 to 46.1 over 12 months[71].

A study of a *Ganoderma lucidum* polysaccharide extract (5.4g/day) showed a 41% reduction in AST values in HBV patients with AST values <100 and a 65% reduction in patients with AST values >100, while ganoderic acid showed significant inhibition of HBV replication, as well as hepatoprotective properties[72,73]. By the end of 6 months 33% of patients had normal AST readings and 13% had cleared hepatitis B surface antigen (HBsAg) from serum whereas none of the controls had normal ALT values or had lost HBsAg.

A number of small Chinese clinical studies report beneficial effects from supplementation with *Cordyceps sinensis* in patients with HBV[74,75,76].

> **CLINICAL NOTE**
>
> *Beneficial results are also reported for C. sinensis biomass in cases of hepatitis C - 2-3g/day.*

Herpes [Tv] [Ps]

In patients with recurrent genital herpes supplementation with 3-5g/day PSK resulted in increased immunity and fewer sick days[77]. *In vitro* research showed PSK to inactivate a laboratory-cultured strain of herpes simplex virus (HSV) type 1 (HSV-1-GC+), together with clinically isolated strains of HSV-2, but found clinically isolated strains of HSV-1 to be resistant[78].

An HSV-1 inhibitory protein has also been reported from *G. frondosa*[79].

CLINICAL NOTE

T. versicolor, or combinations of mushroom polysaccharide extracts help prevent recurrence of HSV outbreaks by maintaining immune competence.

HIV [Cs] [Gl] [Io] [Tv] [Ps]

The nucleoside derivatives found in *Cordyceps sinensis*, including cordycepin (3'-deoxyadenosine), are reverse transcriptase inhibitors of the type now being used to treat HIV and *in vitro* studies confirm them to be effective in inhibiting HIV replication[80-82]. PSK and PSP from *T. versicolor* have also been shown to inhibit both HIV-1 reverse transcriptase and protease, two key enzymes in the life cycle of HIV[83-85], as have triterpenes from *Ganoderma lucidum*, which also inhibit NF-kappaB expression and viral binding[86,87].

There is *in vitro* evidence that betulinic acid analogues (present in *I. obliquus*) disrupt HIV fusion to the cell membrane in a post-binding step through interaction with the viral glycoprotein gp41 as well as disrupting assembly and budding of the HIV-1 virus[88,89], while proteins from *Flammulina velutipes* have been shown to inhibit HIV-1 reverse transcriptase, beta-glucosidase and beta-glucuronidase.

T. versicolor biomass supplementation (3g/day) given as part of traditional Chinese medicine treatment for patients with HIV produced improvements in CD4 count and reductions in viral load as well as fading of Kaposi's sarcoma (caused by human herpes virus 8) in AIDS patients[90,91].

CLINICAL NOTE

C. sinensis shows particular promise in the treatment of HIV and other viral conditions, especially in combination with mushroom polysaccharide extracts.

HPV [Fv] [Tv] [Ps]

In a trial using *Trametes versicolor* biomass (3g/day) 9 of 10 women with high risk strains of HPV had cleared them after 1 year, while only 1 of 12 women in a control group had. Also 13 of 18 patients showed normal cervical cytology after 1 year compared to 10 of 21 in the control group[92].

Supplementation with FVe, a protein from *Flammulina velutipes* significantly enhanced the anti-tumour protection given by vaccination against HPV-16 with the percentage of vaccinated mice remaining tumour free 167 days after challenge with tumour cells increasing from 20% to 60%[93].

> **CLINICAL NOTE**
> *The immune supporting action of mushroom polysaccharides make them ideally suited to assisting with recovery from viral infections such as HPV.*

Hypercholesterolaemia Le Po

Because of their high fibre content, sterols and low calorific value, mushrooms are an ideal food for diets designed to prevent cardiovascular disease and have been extensively investigated for their potential therapeutic application in this regard.

In animal models a range of mushrooms, including *Agaricus bisporus* (common button mushroom), *Grifola frondosa*, *Lentinus edodes*, *Ganoderma lucidum* and *Flammulina velutipes*, all show increased excretion of cholesterol, decreases in LDL and triglycerides and increase in HDL when included in the diet at 5% of feed[94-97]. Similar effects are seen from dietary inclusion of other beta-glucan sources such as oats and barley and it is considered that the action of beta-glucans on cholesterol levels is mediated by their binding affinity for bile acids, leading to activation of cholesterol 7α-hydroxylase and upregulation of low-density lipoprotein receptor and thus increased transportation of LDL into hepatocytes and conversion of cholesterol into bile acids[98].

In addition, some mushrooms show specific cholesterol lowering action. Prominent among these is *Pleurotus ostreatus* (oyster mushroom), which is a natural source of the important cholesterol-lowering drug lovastatin (also called monakolin K, or mevinolin) with higher levels found in the fruiting body (especially in the lamellae or gills) than the mycelium[99].

However, levels of Lovastatin show significant variation from one strain to another making standardised protocols difficult, and better results are achieved clinically with another lovastatin-producing fungus, *Monascus purpureus* (*Hong Qu Mi* - Red Yeast Rice), for which standardised strains are available and for which a much greater impact on cholesterol levels has been demonstrated than achieved by the equivalent dosage of pure lovastatin, implying synergistic action between it and other compounds found in *M. purpureus*.

Eritadenine, a compound isolated from *L. edodes* has demonstrated strong cholesterol lowering properties and it has been suggested that it acts through alteration of hepatic phospholipid metabolism by inhibition of S-adenosylhomocysteine hydrolase, increased excretion and decomposition of ingested cholesterol, and reduced secretion of VLDL by the liver[101]. *L. edodes* fed at 10-50g/kg of diet led to significant decreases in both plasma cholesterol concentration and PC:PE ratio of liver microsomes in rats and eritadenine included at 50mg/kg diet had a similar effect[102].

In clinical trials dried *L. edodes* (9g/day) decreased serum cholesterol 7-10% in patients suffering from hypercholesterolemia and 90g/day fresh *L. edodes* (equivalent to 9g/day dried mushroom) led to a decrease in total cholesterol of 9-12% and triglycerides of 6-7%[103].

Saito et al reported levels of eritadenine of 400-700mg/kg, although Enman et al suggest that the true level may be 10 times greater[104,105]. However, without standardised strains, levels of eritadenine in *L. edodes* are hard to quantify. It has also been shown that stirring rather than shaking during mycelial fermentation can produce a five-fold increase in production of eritadenine, implying significant potential variability in response to cultivation parameters[106].

> **CLINICAL NOTE**
>
> *Two strains of M. purpureus are commercially available, one containing 0.4% lovastatin and the other 0.8%, with clinical trials showing 1200mg/day of the the 0.4% strain to be effective at lowering cholesterol in patients not on prescription statins and 1200mg/day of the 0.8% strain (or 2400mg/day of the 0.4% strain) to be an effective substitute for lovastatin at 10mg/day.*
>
> *Because the eritadenine present in L. edodes works via a different enzymatic pathway from prescription statins or statin containing fungi, it can usefully be combined with them to enhance their impact on cholesterol control.*

Hypertension `Gl`

Ganoderma lucidum has traditionally been used in the treatment of hypertension[107] and ACE inhibitory activity has been demonstrated for the triterpene Ganoderic acid K[108]. It has also been suggested that the CNS inhibiting action of triterpenes from *G. lucidum* may play a part in the anti-hypertensive actions of this mushroom[109].

In the light of recent data, which suggests that subsets of T lymphocytes play critical roles in the development of angiotensin II, deoxycorticosterone salt-sensitive and Dahl salt-sensitive hypertension, and in the progression of vascular remodeling, it is possible that mushrooms may have a beneficial effect on blood pressure by virtue of their immune regulating properties[110].

However, beneficial effects for other mushrooms have only been demonstrated at unrealistic dietary levels of between 5-20%[111-113] or, in the case of *Agaricus brasiliensis*, with a GABA-enriched extract[114].

> **CLINICAL NOTE**
>
> *Triterpene-rich G. lucidum extracts. 1-3g/day.*

Infertility `Cs`

Cordyceps sinensis has a traditional history of use in the treatment of both male and female infertility and *in vitro* studies have shown it to stimulate production of sex hormones through activation of both the protein kinase A and protein kinase C signal transduction pathways[115]. As these pathways are activated by cAMP it is probable that the active component of *C. sinensis* in this regard is one or more of the nucleoside derivatives that it contains.

There is increasing evidence that 17β-estradiol (the predominant form of oestrogen in non-pregnant women) directly influences the quality of maturing oocytes and thus the outcome of assisted reproduction treatment, *C. sinensis* has been shown to upregulate steroidogenic enzymes and ovarian 17β-estradiol (oestrogen) in human granulosa-lutein cells *in vitro*, due, at least in part, to increased StAR and aromatase expression[116]. Ethanolic extracts of *cordyceps* also increased progesterone production in mouse Leydig tumour cells.

In addition, animal studies have shown *C. sinensis* to increase sperm quantity and quality in mouse models[117-119] and *Cordyceps militaris*, a closely related species, to do so in subfertile boars[120].

> **CLINICAL NOTE**
>
> *C. sinensis is an excellent herb for both male and female infertility with 3g/day biomass being a standard dose.*

Inflammatory Bowel Disease (IBD) Tv Gf Ps

As food sources of soluble and insoluble fibre mushrooms and mushroom polysaccharides have been investigated for use in inflammatory bowel disease. In one study whole white button mushroom at 2% of feed exhibited a protective effect[121] while in another beta-glucan from *Pleurotus ostreatus* given at 10% of feed was effective at reducing mucosal damage and myeloperoxidase activity in healthy sections[122]. There is also evidence that supplementation with *Inonotus obliquus* extract can reduce DNA damage in patients with IBD[123].

The ability of chitin to promote wound healing may also have a role to play in helping heal lesions in the intestinal mucosa.

> **CLINICAL NOTE**
>
> *Many of the conditions such as Crohn's Disease and Ulcerative Colitis that fall within the umbrella of IBD are autoimmune in character and hence offer promising targets for the immune modulating action of mushroom polysaccharides. 1-3g/day.*

Influenza Tv Le Ps

Extracts and polysaccharides from different mushrooms, including *Cordyceps sinensis*, *Trametes versicolor*, *Lentinus edodes* and *Grifola frondosa* have been shown to exert an inhibitory effect on influenza virus *in vitro* and *in vivo* through their modulation of immune response[124-127]. Mycelial extracts of edible mushrooms have also been shown to be effective as adjuvants for intranasal influenza vaccine producing a high influenza virus specific IgA and IgG response in nasal washings and serum, respectively[128].

> **CLINICAL NOTE**
>
> *Mushrooms such as T. versicolor and L. edodes can be used prophylactically at the start of the 'flu season' to maintain immune competency, or taken at the onset of symptoms to lessen the duration and severity of colds.*

Insomnia/Anxiety [Gl]

Ganoderma lucidum has traditionally been indicated for the treatment of insomnia[129-131] and aqueous extract from *G. lucidum* fruiting body decreased sleep latency, increased sleeping time, non-REM sleep time and light sleep time in pentobarbital-treated rats in a benzodiazepine-like manner[132].

Clinically, *G. lucidum* is often seen to improve sleep patterns. In his book on medicinal mushrooms Christopher Hobbs reports preferring *G. lucidum* to Valerian for insomnia of a depletion nature[133].

> **CLINICAL NOTE**
>
> *G. lucidum has a subtle but consistent effect on insomnia and anxiety with the triterpenes again the key components. 1-3g/day.*

Kidney Damage [Cs]

Cordyceps sinensis has traditionally been used to strengthen the Kidneys. In one study on 51 patients with chronic renal failure 3-5g/day *C. sinensis* significantly improved kidney function and in another 4.5g/day speeded recovery from gentamycin induced kidney damage with 89% of those taking *C. sinensis* having recovered normal kidney function after 6 days compared to 45% of a control group[134].

> **CLINICAL NOTE**
>
> *With increasing reliance on older, potentially harmful antibiotics to combat multi-resistant strains of bacteria, the ability of C. sinensis to protect the kidneys may assume increasing clinical importance.*

Liver Damage Ac GI Cs

In a study on 14 patients with alcohol induced liver steatosis, supplementation with *Cordyceps sinensis* biomass at 3g/day resulted in a 70% reduction in AST, a 63% reduction in ALT and a 64% reduction in GGT over a 90 day period[135]. Animal studies also show that *C. sinensis* can inhibit alcohol-induced hepatic fibrogenesis, retard the development of cirrhosis and improve liver function[136].

Antrodia camphorata has traditionally been used for the side effects from excess alcohol consumption (including hangovers) and animal studies confirm its ability to protect the liver against chronic alcohol consumption in rats at a dose of 0.1mg/kg[137].

Ganoderma lucidum extracts also demonstrate significant protective action against a range of hepatotoxins, including CCl4, thioacetamide and BCG[138-144].

> **CLINICAL NOTE**
>
> *A. camphorata* and *G. lucidum* are similar in effect and are especially useful where there is active inflammation. Either can also be combined with *C. sinensis* in more chronic situations.

Meniere's Syndrome Am

In China *Armillaria mellea* tablets are prescribed for a range of neurological disorders, including Meniere's Syndrome[145-148].

> **CLINICAL NOTE**
>
> 3-4g/day.

Multiple Sclerosis (MS) He

Together with its ability to promote neuronal repair and regeneration, *in vitro* studies have shown *Hericium erinaceus* to promote nerve myelination, with the process of myelination beginning earlier and proceeding at a higher rate in the presence of *H. erinaceus* extract[149].

> **CLINICAL NOTE**
>
> Although *H. erinaceus* has obvious potential implications for MS, to date no clinical studies have been reported.

Nerve Damage He Gl Tf

Daily administration of aqueous extract of *Hericium erinaceus* fresh fruiting bodies showed a beneficial effect on the recovery of injured rat peroneal nerve in the early stages of regeneration with faster recovery in the treated group than in the untreated group[150].

G. lucidum spores have also shown beneficial activity in a mouse nerve damage model while *Tremella fuciformis* polysaccharides increased neurite outgrowth in PC12 cells, indicating potential to promote NGF production[151].

> **CLINICAL NOTE**
>
> *H. erinaceus 3-5g/day dried fruit body can be combined with T. fuciformis polysaccharides or G. lucidum sporoderm-broken spores.*

Parkinsons Disease (PD) Fv Gl

Several papers report increased levels of pro-inflammatory cytokines such as tumour necrosis factor (TNF)-alpha, IL-1beta and IL-6, and decreased levels of neurotrophins such as brain-derived neurotrophic factor (BDNF) in patients with sporadic PD, with the possibility that the ability of mushroom polysaccharides to promote a shift in immune response away from a pro-inflammatory Th2 cytokine profile to a Th1 dominant state may be of benefit to patients with early stage PD[152].

The tyrosinase inhibiting activity of mushrooms like *Ganoderma lucidum* and *Flammulina velutipes* may also play a role in controlling the development of PD. Tyrosinase catalyses the oxidation of tyrosine and dopamine, producing dopaquinone, which besides being the common precursor of the different forms of melanin, is a dopaminergic neuron-specific cytotoxic molecule[153,154]. Dopaquinone can also covalently modify and inactivate tyrosine hydroxylase, the rate limiting enzyme in catecholamine biosynthesis, leading to further reductions in levels of dopamine[155].

In addition tyrosinase contributes to the formation of neuromelanin, which identifies neurons susceptible to Parkinson's disease in cell culture systems and has been implicated in the development of the disease[156].

> **CLINICAL NOTE**
>
> *Culinary mushrooms such as F. velutipes are usually preferred for long term supplementation in chronic conditions like PD.*

Rheumatoid Arthritis (RA)

A polysaccharide extract from the fruiting body of *Phellinus linteus* reduced expression of pro-inflammatory cytokines and increased expression of anti-inflammtory cytokines, resulting in subsidence of the autoimmune response in the joints of mice[157]. Fungal polysaccharides have also been shown to reduce inflammation and have a positive modulating effect on plasma cytokine levels[158] in experimentally induced arthritis in rats, while the triterpenes from *Ganoderma lucidum* exhibit strong anti-inflammatory action[159,160].

CLINICAL NOTE

While mushroom polysaccharides, such as those from P. linteus, are excellent for promoting a shift away from the Th2 cytokine profile characteristic of RA, the stronger anti-inflammatory properties of triterpene-rich G. lucidum extracts are better suited to use during more active phases.

Systemic Lupus Erythematosus (SLE)

A mycelial extract of *Antrodia camphorata* reduced urine protein and creatinine levels and suppressed the thickening of the kidney glomerular basement membrane at 400mg/kg in a mouse model of SLE, suggesting ability to protect the kidney from immunological damage resulting from autoimmune disease[161].

REFERENCES

1. Anti-allergic constituents in the culture medium of *Ganoderma lucidum*. (I). Inhibitory effect of oleic acid on histamine release. Tasaka K, Akagi M, Miyoshi K, Mio M, Makino T. Inflammation Research. 1988;23(3-4):153-6
2. Anti-allergic constituents in the culture medium of *Ganoderma lucidum*. (II). The inhibitory effect of cyclooctasulfur on histamine release. Tasaka K, Mio M, Izushi K, Akagi M, Makino T. Inflammation Research. 1988;23(3-4):157-60
3. Effectiveness of Dp2 nasal therapy for Dp2- induced airway inflammation in mice: using oral *Ganoderma lucidum* as an immunomodulator. Liu Y.H, Tsai C.F, Kao M.C, Lai Y.L, Tsai J.J. J Microbiol Immunol Infect. 2003;36(4):236-428
4. The use of *Ganoderma lucidum* (Reishi) in the management of Histamine-mediated allergic responses. Powell M. Nutritional Practitioner Magazine. October 2004
5. Antagonizing beta-amyloid peptide neurotoxicity of the anti-aging fungus *Ganoderma lucidum*. Lai C.S, Yu M.S, Yuen W.H, So K.F, Zee S.Y, Chang R.C. Brain Res. 2008;1190:215-24
6. Medicinal value of the caterpillar fungi species of the genus *Cordyceps*. Holliday J, Cleaver M. Int J Med Mushr. 2008;10(3):219-234
7. Effect of dongchong xiacao capsule on airway inflammation of asthmatic patients. Wang N.Q, Jiang L.D, Zhang X.M, Li Z.X. Zhongguo Zhong Yao Za Zhi. 2007;32(15):1566-8
8. Effects of fermented *Cordyceps* powder on pulmonary function in sensitized guinea pigs and airway inflammation in sensitized rats. Lin X.X, Xie Q.M, Shen W.H, Chen Y. Zhongguo Zhong Yao Za Zhi. 2001;26(9):622-5
9. Effects of *Cordyceps sinensis*, *Cordyceps militaris* and their isolated compounds on ion transport in Calu-3 human airway epithelial cells. Yue G.G, Lau C.B, Fung K, Leung P, Ko W. Journal of Ethnopharmacology. 2008;117(1):92-1014
10. Regulation of bronchoalveolar lavage fluids cell function by the immunomodulatory agents from *Cordyceps sinensis*. Kuo Y.C, Tsai W.J, Wang J.Y, Chang S.C, Lin C.Y, Shiao M.S. Life Sci. 2001;68(9):1067-82
11. *Ganoderma tsugae* supplementation alleviates bronchoalveolar inflammation in an airway sensitization and challenge mouse model. Lin J.Y, Chen M.L, Chiang B.L, Lin B.F. Int Immunopharmacol. 2006;6(2):241-51
12. Effects of triterpenoid-rich extracts of *Ganoderma tsugae* on airway hyperreactivity and Th2 responses *in vivo*. Chen M.L, Lin B.F. Int Arch Allergy Immunol. 2007;143(1):21-30
13. Amelioration of skewed Th1/Th2 balance in tumour-bearing and asthma-induced mice by oral administration of *Agaricus blazei* extracts. Takimoto H, Kato H, Kaneko M, Kumazawa Y. Immunopharmacol Immunotoxicol. 2008;30(4):747-60

14. Potential of the beta-glucans to enhance innate resistance to biological agents. Thompson I.J, Oyston P.C, Williamson D.E. Expert Rev Anti Infect Ther. 2010;8(3):339-52

15. An examination of antibacterial and antifungal properties of constituents of Shiitake (*Lentinula edodes*) and oyster (*Pleurotus ostreatus*) mushrooms. Hearst R, Nelson D, McCollum G, Millar B.C, Maeda Y, Goldsmith C.E, Rooney P.J, Loughrey A, Rao J.R, Moore J.E. Complement Ther Clin Pract. 2009;15(1):5-7

16. Screening of Basidiomycetes for antimicrobial activities. Suay I, Arenal F. Antonie van Leeuwenhoek 2000;78:129-139

17. Anti-MRSA compounds of *Hericium erinaceus*. Kawagishi H et al. Int J Med Mushr. 2005;7(3):350

18. Two cyathane-type diterpenoids from the liquid culture of *Strobilurus tenacellus*. Shiono Y, Hiramatsu F, Murayama T, Koseki T, Funakoshi T. Chem Biodivers. 2008;5(9):1811-6

19. Anti-androgenic activities of *Ganoderma lucidum*. Fujita R, Liu J, Shimizu K, Konishi F, Noda K, Kumamoto S, Ueda C, Tajiri H, Kaneko S, Suimi Y, Kondo R. J Ethnopharmacol. 2005; 102(1):107-12

20. The anti-androgen effect of ganoderol B isolated from the fruiting body of Ganoderma lucidum. Liu J, Shimizu K, Konishi F, Kumamoto S, Kondo R. Bioorg Med Chem. 2007; 15(14):4966-72

21. Structure-activity relationship for inhibition of 5alpha-reductase by triterpenoids isolated from *Ganoderma lucidum*. Liu J, Kurashiki K, Shimizu K, Kondo R. Bioorg Med Chem. 2006; 14(24):8654-60

22. 5alpha-reductase inhibitory effect of triterpenoids isolated from *Ganoderma lucidum*. Liu J, Kurashiki K, Shimizu K, Kondo R. Biol Pharm Bull. 2006;29(2):392-5

23. Antifungal secondary metabolites from fungal fruiting bodies. Dunek C, Volk T.J. Int J Med Mushr. 2007;9(3):227-228

24. An examination of antibacterial and antifungal properties of constituents of Shiitake (*Lentinula edodes*) and oyster (*Pleurotus ostreatus*) mushrooms. Hearst R, Nelson D, McCollum G, Millar B.C, Maeda Y, Goldsmith C.E, Rooney P.J, Loughrey A, Rao J.R, Moore J.E. Complement Ther Clin Pract. 2009;15(1):5-7

25. Antimicrobial properties of shiitake mushrooms (*Lentinula edodes*). Rao J.R, Smyth T.J, Millar B.C, Moore J.E. Int J Antimicrob Agents. 2009;33(6):591-2

26. Antagonistic effect of edible mushroom extract on *Candia albicans* growth. Paccola E, Maki C.S, Nobrega G.M.A, Paccola-Meirelles L.D. Braz J Microbiol. 2001;32:3

27. Antimicrobial and antineoplasic activity of *Pleurotus ostreatus*. Wolff E.R, Wisbeck E, Silveira M.L, Gern R.M, Pinho M.S, Furlan S.A. Appl Biochem Biotechnol. 2008;151(2-3):402-12

28. Antimicrobial action of *Lentinus edodes* juice on human microflora. Kuznetsov O.I, Mil'kova E.V, Sosnina A.E, Sotnikova N.I. Zh Mikrobiol Epidemiol Immunobiol. 2005; 1:80-2

29. Polysaccharide-rich fraction of *Agaricus brasiliensis* enhances the candidacidal activity of murine macrophages. Martins P.R, Gameiro M.C, Castoldi L, Romagnoli G.G, Lopes F.C, Pinto A.V, Loyola W, Kaneno R. Mem Inst Oswaldo Cruz. 2008;103(3):244-50

30. Fungal Chitin in medicine: prospects for its application. Ludmila I.B, Leontij F.G. Int J Med Mushr. 2001;3(2-3)126-127

31. Protective effects of a protein-bound polysaccharide, PSK, on Candida albicans infection in mice via tumour necrosis factor-alpha induction. Ohmura Y, Matsunaga K, Motokawa I, Sakurai K, Ando T. Int Immunopharmacol. 2001;1:1797-1811

32. Protective effects of a protein-bound polysaccharide, PSK, against Candida albicans infection in syngeneic tumour-bearing mice via Th1 cell functions. Ohmura Y, Matsunaga K, Motokawa I, Sakurai K, Ando T. Cancer Biother Radiopharm. 2003;18(5):769-80

33. A formal analysis of cytokine networks in Chronic Fatigue Syndrome. Broderick G, Fuite J, Kreitz A, Vernon S.D, Klimas N, Fletcher M.A. Brain Behav Immun. 2010;24(7):1209-17

34. Plasma cytokines in women with chronic fatigue syndrome. Fletcher M.A, Zeng X.R, Barnes Z, Levis S, Klimas N.G. J Transl Med. 2009;7:96

35. High levels of type 2 cytokine-producing cells in chronic fatigue syndrome. Skowera A, Cleare A, Blair D, Bevis L, Wessely S.C, Peakman M. Clin Exp Immunol. 2004;135(2):294-302

36. Pioneering work at breakspear hospital on *Coriolus* Supplementation for CFIDS/ME patients. Mycology News. 2000;1(4):4

37. Improving effects of the mushroom Yamabushitake (*Hericium erinaceus*) on mild cognitive impairment: a double-blind placebo-controlled clinical trial. Mori K, Inatomi S, Ouchi K, Azumi Y, Tuchida T. Phytother Res. 2009;23(3):367-72

38. The anti-Dementia effect of Lion's mane mushroom and its clinical application. Kawagishi H, Zhuang C, Shnidman E. Townsend Letter for Doctors and Patients. April, 2004

39. Beta-glucans in the treatment of diabetes and associated cardiovascular risks. Chen J, Raymond K. Vasc Health Risk Manag. 2008;4(6):1265-72

40. A controlled study of consumption of beta-glucan-enriched soups for 2 months by type 2 diabetic free-living subjects. Cugnet-Anceau C, Nazare J.A, Biorklund M, Le Coquil E, Sassolas A, Sothier M, Holm J, Landin-Olsson M, Onning G, Laville M, Moulin P. Br J Nutr. 2010;103(3):422-8

41. The mushroom *Agaricus Blazei* Murill in combination with metformin and gliclazide improves insulin resistance in type 2 diabetes: a randomized, double-blinded, and placebo-controlled clinical trial. Hsu C.H, Liao Y.L, Lin S.C, Hwang K.C, Chou P. J Altern Complement Med. 2007;13(1):97-102

42. Hypoglycemic effect of water-soluble polysaccharide from Auricularia auricula-judae Quel. on genetically diabetic KK-Ay mice. Yuan Z, He P, Cui J, Takeuchi H. Biosci Biotechnol Biochem. 1998;62(10):1898-903

43. Clinical observations of adjunctive treatment of 20 diabetic patients with JinShuiBao capsule. Guo Q.C, Zhang C, Lo H.C, Tu S.T, Lin K.C, Lin S.C. J Admin Trad Chin Med. 1995; 5:223

44. The anti-hyperglycemic activity of the fruiting body of *Cordyceps* in diabetic rats induced by nicotinamide and streptozotocin. Life Sci. 2004;74(23):2897-908

45. CordyMax Cs-4 improves glucose metabolism and increases insulin sensitivity in normal rats. Zhao C.S, Yin W.T, Wang J.Y, Zhang Y, Yu H, Cooper R, Smidt C, Zhu J.S. J Altern Complement Med. 2002;8(3):309-14.7

46. A phase I/II study of Ling Zhi mushroom *Ganoderma lucidum* (W.Curt.:Fr.)Lloyd (Aphyllophoromycetideae) extract in patients with type II Diabetes mellitus. Gao Y, Lan J, Dai X, Ye J, Zhou S. Int J Med Mushr. 2004;6(1)

47. A randomized, double-blind and placebo-controlled study of a *Ganoderma lucidum* polysaccharide extract in neurasthenia. Tang W, Gao Y, Chen G, Gao H, Dai X, Ye J, Chan E, Huang M, Zhou S. J Med Food. 2005;8(1):53-8

48. Anti-diabetic activity present in the fruit body of *Grifola frondosa* (Maitake). Kubo K, Aoki H, Nanba H. I. Biol Pharm Bull. 1994;17(8):1106-10

49. Maitake (*Grifola frondosa*) improve glucose tolerance of experimental diabetic rats. Horio H, Ohtsuru M. J Nutr Sci Vitaminol (Tokyo). 2001;47(1):57-63

50. Antihypertensive and metabolic effects of whole Maitake mushroom powder and its fractions in two rat strains. Talpur N.A, Echard B.W, Fan A.Y, Jaffari O, Bagchi D, Preuss H.G. Mol Cell Biochem. 2002;237(1-2):129-36

51. Hypoglycemic effect of extract of *Hericium erinaceus*. Wang J.C, Hu S.H, Wang J.T, Chen K.S, Chia Y.C. Journal of the Science of Food and Agriculture. 2005;85(4):641-646

52. Effect of the oyster fungus on glycaemia and cholesterolaemia in rats with insulin-dependent diabetes. Chorváthová V, Bobek P, Ginter E, Klvanová J. Physiol Res. 1993;42(3):175-9

53. Oyster mushroom reduced blood glucose and cholesterol in diabetic subjects. Khatun K, Mahtab H, Khanam P.A, Sayeed M.A, Khan K.A. Mymensingh Med J. 2007;16(1):94-9

54. Hypoglycemic effects of exopolysaccharides produced by mycelial cultures of two different mushrooms *Tremella fuciformis* and Phellinus baumii in ob/ob mice. Cho E.J, Hwang H.J, Kim S.W, Oh J.Y, Baek Y.M, Choi J.W, Bae S.H, Yun J.W. Appl Microbiol Biotechnol. 2007;75(6):1257-65

55. Effect of *Coprinus comatus* on plasma Glucose concentrations in mice. Bailey C.J, Turner S.L, Jakeman K.J, Hayes W.A. Planta Med. 1984;50(6):525-526

56. Vanadium uptake by biomass of *Coprinus comatus* and their effect on hyperglycemic mice. Han C, Cui B, Wang Y. Biol Trace Elem Res. 2008;124(1):35-9

57. Comparison of vanadium-rich activity of three species fungi of basidiomycetes. Han C, Cui B, Qu J. Biol Trace Elem Res. 2009;127(3):278-83

58. Comparison of hypoglycemic activity of trace elements absorbed in fermented mushroom of *Coprinus comatus*. Lv Y, Han L, Yuan C, Guo J. Biol Trace Elem Res. 2009;131(2):177-85

59. Han C, Yuan J, Wang Y, Li L. Hypoglycemic activity of fermented mushroom of *Coprinus comatus* rich in vanadium. J Trace Elem Med Biol. 2006;20(3):191-6

60. Determination of trace elements in three mushroom samples of Basidiomycetes from Shandong, China. Wang C, Hou Y. Biol Trace Elem Res. 2010 Jul 28

61. Regulatory mechanism of *Cordyceps sinensis* mycellium on mouse Leydig cell steroidogenesis. Hsu C.C, Tsai S.J, Huang Y.L, Huang B.M. FEBS Lett. 2003;543(1-3):140-3

62. The *in vivo* effect of *Cordyceps sinensis* mycelium on plasma corticosterone level in male mouse. Leu S.F, Chien C.H, Tseng C.Y, Kuo Y.M, Huang B.M. Biol Pharm Bull. 2005;28(9):1722-5

63. Regulation of steroidogenesis by *Cordyceps sinensis* mycelium extracted fractions with (hCG) treatment in mouse Leydig cells. Wong K.L, So E.C, Chen C.C, Wu R.S, Huang B.M. Arch Androl. 2007;53(2):75-7

64. An anti-aldosteronic diuretic component (drain dampness) in *Polyporus sclerotium*. Yuan D, et al. Biol Pharm Bull. 2004;27(6):867-70

65. Bioactivity-directed isolation, identification of diuretic compounds from *Polyporus umbellatus*. Zhao Y.Y, Xie R.M, Chao X, Zhang Y, Lin R.C, Sun W.J. J Ethnopharmacol. 2009;126(1):184-7

66. A double-blind study of effectiveness of *Hericium erinaceus* pers therapy on chronic atrophic gastritis. A preliminary report. Xu C.P, Liu W.W, Liu F.X, Chen S.S, Liao F.Q, Xu Z, Jiang L.G, Wang C.A, Lu X.H. Chin Med J (Engl). 1985;98(6):455-6

67. Cytoprotective effects of *Hericium erinaceus* on gastric mucosa in rats. Yu C.G, Xu Z.M, Zhu Q.K et al. Chinese J Gastrent. 1999-02

68. Effect of culinary-medicinal Lion's Mane mushroom, *Hericium erinaceus* (Bull.: Fr.) Pers. (Aphyllophoromycetideae), on Ethanol-induced gastric ulcers in rats. Abdulla M.A, Noor S, Sabaratnam V, Abdullah N, Wong K.H, Ali H.M. Int J Med Mush. 2008;10(4):325-330

69. Clinical and experimental research on *Polyporus umbellatus* polysaccharide in the treatment of chronic viral hepatitis. Yan SC, Zhong Xi Yi Jie He Za Zhi. 1988;8(3):141-3, 131

70. Chinese medicinal herbs for chronic hepatitis B: a systematic review. Liver. Liu J, McIntosh H, Lin H. 2001;21(4):280-6

71. The mushroom *Agaricus blazei* Murill extract normalizes liver function in patients with chronic hepatitis B. Hsu C.H, Hwang K.C, Chiang Y.H, Chou P. J Altern Complement Med. 2008; 14(3):299-301

72. A phase I/II study of a *Ganoderma lucidum* (Curt.: Fr.) P. Karst. (Ling Zhi, Reishi Mushroom) extract in patients with chronic Hepatitis B. Gao Y, Zhou S, Chen G, Dai X, Ye J, Gao H. Int J Med Mush. 2002

73. Anti-hepatitis B activities of ganoderic acid from *Ganoderma lucidum*. Li Y.Q, Wang S.F. Biotechnol Lett. 2006;28(11):837-41

74. Short-term curative effect of cultured *Cordyceps sinensis* (Berk.) Sacc. Mycelia in chronic hepatitis B. Zhou L, Yang W, Xu Y, Zhu Q, Ma Z, Zhu T, Ge X, Gao J. Zhongguo Zhong Yao Za Zhi. 1990;15(1):53-5, 65

75. Effects of *Cordyceps* polysaccharides in patients with chronic hepatitis C. X Ma, D.K Qiu, J Xu, M.D Zeng. Huaren Xiaohua Zazhi 1998;6:582-584 6

76. Effects of *cordyceps sinensis* on T lymphocyte subsets and hepato-fibrosis in patients with chronic hepatitis B. Gong H.Y, Wang K.Q, Tang S.G. Hunan Yi Ke Da Xue Xue Bao. 2000;25(3):248-50

77. Treatment of recurrent genital herpes with PSK. Kawana T. Proceedings of the International Symposium on Pharmacological and Clinical Approaches to Herpes Viruses and Virus Chemotherapy. Oiso, Japan, Sept. 10-13, 1984

78. in vitro inactivation of herpes simplex virus by a biological response modifier, PSK. Monma Y, Kawana T, Shimizu F. Antiviral Res. 1997;35(3):131-8

79. Isolation, identification and function of a novel anti-HSV-1 protein from *Grifola frondosa*. Gu C.Q, Li J.W, Chao F, Jin M, Wang X.W, Shen Z.Q. Antiviral Res. 2007;75(3):250-7

80. Emerging antiviral drugs from medicinal mushrooms. Pirano F.F. Int J Med Mushr. 2006;8(2):20

81. Phosphorothioate and cordycepin analogues of 2', 5'-oligoadenylate: Inhibition of human immunodeficiency virus type 1 reverse transcriptase and infection *in vitro*. We Robinson Jr et al. Proc Natl Acad Sci USA. 1989;86: 7191-7194

82. Synthesis, characterization, and biological activity of monomeric and trimeric cordycepin-cholesterol conjugates and inhibition of HIV-1 replication. Wasner M, Henderson E.E, Suhadolnik R.J, Pfleiderer W. Helvetica Chimica Acta. 1994;77:1757-1761

83. Polysaccharopeptide from the Turkey tail fungus *Trametes versicolor* (L.:Fr.) Pilát inhibits human immunodeficiency virus type 1 reverse Transciptase and Protease. Ng T.B, Wang H.X, Wan D.C.C. Int J Med Mushr. 2006;8(1):40

84. Polysaccharopeptide from *Coriolus versicolor* has potential for use against human immunodeficiency virus type 1 infection. Collins R.A, Ng T.B. Life Sci. 1997;60(25):383-7

85. A biological response modifier, PSK, inhibits reverse transcriptase *in vitro*. Hirose K, Hakozaki M, Kakuchi J, Matsunaga K, Yoshikumi C, Takahashi M, Tochikura T.S, Yamamoto N. Biochem Biophys Res Commun. 1987;149(2):562-7

86. Anti-HIV-1 and anti-HIV-1-protease substances from *Ganoderma lucidum*. el-Mekkawy S, Meselhy M.R, Nakamura N, Tezuka Y, Hattori M, Kakiuchi N, Shimotohno K, Kawahata T, Otake T. Phytochemistry. 1998;49(6):1651-7

87. Triterpenes from the spores of *Ganoderma lucidum* and their inhibitory activity against HIV-1 protease. Min B.S, Nakamura N, Miyashiro H, Bae K.W, Hattori M. Chem Pharm Bull (Tokyo). 1998;46(10):1607-12

88. Chemistry, biological activity, and chemotherapeutic potential of betulinic acid for the prevention and treatment of cancer and HIV infection. Cichewicz R.H, Kouzi S.A. Med Res Rev. 2004;24(1):90-114

89. Betulinic acid derivatives as human immunodeficiency virus type 2 (HIV-2) inhibitors. Dang Z, Lai W, Qian K, Ho P, Lee K.H, Chen C.H, Huang L. J Med Chem. 2009; 52(23):7887-91

90. The effectiveness of *Coriolus versicolor* supplementation in the treatment of Kaposi sarcoma in HIV+Patients. Tindall J, Clegg E. Presented at the 10th International Congress of Mucosal Immunology in Amsterdam, June 28th - July 1st, 1999

91. The clinical use of *Coriolus versicolor* supplementation in HIV+ patients and the impact on CD4 count and viral load. Pfeiffer M. Presented at the III International Symposium on Mushroom Nutrition in Milan on Saturday, March 10th, 2001

92. *Coriolus versicolor* supplementation in HPV patients. Dr. Jose Silva Couto and Dr. Daniel Pereira da Silva. 20th European Congress of Obstetrics and Gynaecology. March 7th, 2008

93. Coadministration of the fungal immunomodulatory protein FIP-Fve and a tumour-associated antigen enhanced antitumour immunity. Ding Y, Seow S.V, Huang C.H, Liew L.M, Lim Y.C, Kuo I.C, Chua K.Y. Immunology. 2009;128(1Suppl):e881-94

94. White button mushroom (*Agaricus bisporus*) lowers blood glucose and cholesterol levels in diabetic and hypercholesterolemic rats. Jeong S.C, Jeong Y.T, Yang B.K, Islam R, Koyyalamudi S.R, Pang G, Cho K.Y, Song C.H. Nutr Res. 2010;30(1):49-56

95. Cholesterol-lowering effects of maitake (*Grifola frondosa*) fiber, shiitake (*Lentinus edodes*) fiber, and enokitake (*Flammulina velutipes*) fiber in rats. Fukushima M, Ohashi T, Fujiwara Y, Sonoyama K, Nakano M. Exp Biol Med (Maywood). 2001;226(8):758-65

96. Maitake extracts and their therapeutic potential - A Review. Mayell M. Alt Med Rev, 2001;6:1

97. Cholesterol-lowering properties of *Ganoderma lucidum in vitro, ex-vivo*, and in hamsters and minipigs. Berger A, Rein D, Kratky E, Monnard I, Piguet-Welsch C, Hauser J, Mace K, Niederberger P. Lipids in Health and Disease 2004;3:2

98. Effect of high beta-glucan barley on serum cholesterol concentrations and visceral fat area in Japanese men - A randomised, double-blinded, placebo controlled trial. Shimizu C, Kihara M, Aoe S et al. Plant Foods Hum Nutr. 2008;63:21-5

99. *Pleurotus* fruiting bodies contain the inhibitor of 3-hydroxy-3-methyl-glutaryl-coenzyme A reductase - lovastatin. Gunde-Cimerman N, Cimerman A. Exp Mycol. 1995;19(1):1-6

100. Dose and time dependent hypercholesterolemic effect of oyster mushroom (*Pleurotus ostreatus*) in rats. Nutrition. 1998;14:282-286

101. Eritadenine-induced alterations of plasma lipoprotein lipid concentrations and phosphatidylcholine molecular species profile in rats fed cholesterol-free and cholesterol-enriched diets. Shimada Y, Morita T, Sugiyama K. Biosci Biotechnol Biochem. 2003 May;67(5):996-1006

102. Hypocholesterolemic action of eritadenine is mediated by a modification of hepatic phospholipid metabolism in rats. Sugiyama K, Akachi T, Yamakawa A. J Nutr. 1995;125(8):2134-44

103. Shiitake (*Lentinus edodes*) Wasser S.P. Encyclopedia of Dietary Supplements. 2005

104. Quantitative analysis of eritadenine in "Shii-take" mushroom and other edible fungi. Saito M, Yamashita T, Kaneda T. Eiyo to Shokuryo. Pub Informa Healthcare. 1975;28:503-505

105. Quantification of the bioactive compound eritadenine in selected strains of shiitake mushroom (*Lentinus edodes*). Enman J, Rova U, Berglund K.A. J Agric Food Chem. 2007;55(4):1177-80

106. Production of the bioactive compound eritadenine by submerged cultivation of shiitake (*Lentinus edodes*) mycelia. Enman J, Hodge D, Berglund K.A, Rova U.J. Agric Food Chem. 2008;56(8):2609-12

107. Dietary effect of *Ganoderma lucidum* mushroom on blood pressure and lipid levels in spontaneously hypertensive rats (SHR). Kabir Y, Kimura S, Tamura T. J Nutr Sci Vitaminol (Tokyo). 1988;34(4):433-8

108. Effect of *Ganoderma lucidum* on the quality and functionality of Korean traditional rice wine, yakju. Kim J.H, Lee D.H, Lee S.H, Choi S.Y, Lee J.S. J Biosci Bioeng. 2004;97(1):24-8

109. Cardiovascular effects of mycelium extract of *Ganoderma lucidum*: inhibition of sympathetic outflow as a mechanism of its hypotensive action. Lee S.Y, Rhee H.M. Chem Pharm Bull (Tokyo). 1990;38(5):1359-64

110. T lymphocytes: a role in hypertension? Schiffrin E.L. Curr Opin Nephrol Hypertens. 2010;19(2):181-6

111. Effect of shiitake (*Lentinus edodes*) and maitake (*Grifola frondosa*) mushrooms on blood pressure and plasma lipids of spontaneously hypertensive rats. Kabir Y, Yamaguchi M, Kimura S. J Nutr Sci Vitaminol (Tokyo). 1987;33(5):341-6

112. Antihypertensive and metabolic effects of whole Maitake mushroom powder and its fractions in two rat strains. Talpur N.A, Echard B.W, Fan A.Y, Jaffari O, Bagchi D, Preuss H.G. Mol Cell Biochem. 2002;237(1-2):129-36.3

113. Dietary mushrooms reduce blood pressure in spontaneously hypertensive rats (SHR). Kabir Y, Kimura S. J Nutr Sci Vitaminol (Tokyo). 1989;35(1):91-4

114. Watanabe T, Kawashita A, Ishi S, Mazumder T.K, Nagai S, Tsuji K, Dan T. Antihypertensive effect of γ-aminobutyric acid-enriched *Agaricus blazei* on mild hypertensive human subjects. Nippon Shokuhin Kagaku Kogaku Kaishi. 2003;50(4):167-173

115. *Cordyceps sinensis* mycelium activates PKA and PKC signal pathways to stimulate steroidogenesis in MA-10 mouse Leydig tumour cells. Chen Y.C, Huang Y.L, Huang B.M. Int J Biochem Cell Biol. 2005;37(1):214-23

116. Upregulation of steroidogenic enzymes and ovarian 17beta-estradiol in human granulosa-lutein cells by *Cordyceps sinensis* mycelium. Huang B.M, Hsiao K.Y, Chuang P.C, Wu M.H, Pan H.A, Tsai S.J. Biol Reprod. 2004;70(5):1358-64

117. Regulation of steroidogenesis by *Cordyceps sinensis* mycelium extracted fractions with (hCG) treatment in mouse Leydig cells. Wong K.L, So E.C, Chen C.C, Wu R.S, Huang B.M. Arch Androl. 2007;53(2):75-7

118. Regulatory mechanism of *Cordyceps sinensis* mycellium on mouse Leydig cell steroidogenesis. Hsu C.C, Tsai S.J, Huang Y.L, Huang B.M. FEBS Lett. 2003;543(1-3):140-3

119. *in vivo* stimulatory effect of *Cordyceps sinensis* mycelium and its fractions on reproductive functions in male mouse. Huang Y.L, Leu S.F, Liu B.C, Sheu C.C, Huang B.M. Life Sci. 2004;75(9):1051-62119

120. Improvement of sperm production in subfertile boars by *Cordyceps militaris* supplement. Lin W.H, Tsai M.T, Chen Y.S, Hou R.C, Hung H.F, Li C.H, Wang H.K, Lai M.N, Jeng K.C. Am J Chin Med. 2007;35(4):631-41

121. The effects of whole mushrooms during inflammation. Yu S, Weaver V, Martin K, Cantorna M.T. BMC Immunol. 2009;10:12

122. Effects of pleuran (beta-glucan isolated from *Pleurotus ostreatus*) on experimental colitis in rats. Nosál'ová V, Bobek P, Cerná S, Galbavý S, Stvrtina S. Physiol Res. 2001;50(6):575-81

123. Chaga mushroom extract inhibits oxidative DNA damage in lymphocytes of patients with inflammatory bowel diseas. Najafzadeh M, Reynolds P.D, Baumgartner A, Jerwood D, Anderson D. Biofactors. 2007;31(3-4):191-200

124. *in vivo* anti-influenza virus activity of an immunomodulatory acidic polysaccharide isolated from *Cordyceps militaris* grown on germinated soybeans. Ohta Y, Lee J.B, Hayashi K, Fujita A, Park D.K, Hayashi T. J Agric Food Chem. 2007;55(25):10194-9

125. Inhibitory effect of TNF-alpha produced by macrophages stimulated with *Grifola frondosa* extract (ME) on the growth of influenza A/Aichi/2/68 virus in MDCK cells. Obi N, Hayashi K, Miyahara T, Shimada Y, Terasawa K, Watanabe M, Takeyama M, Obi R, Ochiai H. Am J Chin Med. 2008;36(6):1171-83

126. Antiviral and interferon-inducing activities of a new peptidomannan, KS-2, extracted from culture mycelia of *Lentinus edodes*. Suzuki F, Suzuki C, Shimomura E, Maeda H, Fujii T, Ishida N. J Antibiot (Tokyo). 1979;32(12):1336-45

127. Depression of early protection against influenza virus infection by cyclophosphamide and its restoration by protein-bound polysaccharide. Tsuru S. Kitasato Arch Exp Med. 1992;65(2-3):97-110

128. Induction of cross-protective immunity against influenza A virus H5N1 by an intranasal vaccine with extracts of mushroom mycelia. Ichinohe T, Ainai A, Nakamura T, Akiyama Y, Maeyama J, Odagiri T, Tashiro M, Takahashi H, Sawa H, Tamura S, Chiba J, Kurata T, Sata T, Hasegawa H. J Med Virol. 2010;82(1):128-37

129. Sleep-promoting effects of *Ganoderma* extracts in rats: comparison between long-term and acute administrations. Honda K, Komoda Y, Inoué S. Tokyo Ika Shika Daigaku Iyo Kizai Kenkyusho Hokoku. 1988;22:77-82

130. The hypnotic and sedative actions of the spores of *Ganoderma lucidum* (Curt.: Fr.) P. Karst. (Aphyllophoromycetideae) in mice. Yu L, Wei H. Int J Med Mushr. 2000;2(4):323-328

131. *Ganoderma lucidum*: a potent pharmacological macrofungus. Sanodiya B.S, Thakur G.S, Baghel R.K, Prasad G.B, Bisen P.S. Curr Pharm Biotechnol. 2009;10(8):717-42

132. Extract of *Ganoderma lucidum* potentiates pentobarbital-induced sleep via a GABAergic mechanis. Chu Q.P, Wang L.E, Cui X.Y, Fu H.Z, Lin Z.B, Lin S.Q, Zhang Y.H. Pharmacology Biochemistry and Behavior. 2007;86(4):693-698

133. Hobbs C. Medicinal Mushrooms: An Exploration of Tradition, Healing and Culture. 1986 Botanica Press, Williams

134. Medicinal value of the caterpillar fungi species of the *genus Cordyceps* (Fr.) link (Ascomycetes). A Review. Holliday J, Cleaver M. Int J Med Mush. 2008;10(3):219–234

135. *Cordyceps sinensis* supplementation in alcohol-induced liver steatosis. Santos C. Mycology News, 2004;1(9)

136. Inhibitive effect of *Cordyceps sinensis* on experimental hepatic fibrosis and its possible mechanism. Liu Y.K, Shen W. World J Gastroenterol. 2003;9(3):529-33

137. Fruiting body of Niuchangchih (*Antrodia camphorata*) protects livers against chronic alcohol consumption damage. Huang C.H, Chang Y.Y, Liu C.W, Kang W.Y, Lin Y.L, Chang H.C, Chen Y.C. J Agric Food Chem. 2010;58(6):3859-66

138. Effect of polysaccharide peptide (PSP) on glutathione and protection against paracetamol-induced hepatotoxicity in the rat. Yeung J.H, Chiu L.C, Ooi V.E. Methods Find Exp Clin Pharmacol. 1994;16(10):723-9

139. Immunopharmacologic agents in the amelioration of hepatic injuries. Farghali H, Masek K. Int J Immunopharmacol. 1998;20(4-5):125-39

140. Beta-glucuronidase-inhibitory activity and hepatoprotective effect of *Ganoderma lucidum*. Kim D.H, Shim S.B, Kim N.J, Jang I.S. Biol Pharm Bull. 1999;22(2):162-4

141. Evaluation of the hepatic and renal-protective effects of *Ganoderma lucidum* in mice. Shieh Y.H, Liu C.F, Huang Y.K, Yang J.Y, Wu I.L, Lin C.H, Li S.C. Am J Chin Med. 2001;29(3-4):501-7

142. Hepatoprotective role of *Ganoderma lucidum* polysaccharide against BCG-induced immune liver injury in mice. Zhang G.L, Wang Y.H, Ni W, Teng H.L, Lin Z.B. World J Gastroenterol. 2002;8(4):728-33

143. Protection against D-galactosamine-induced acute liver injury by oral administration of extracts from *Lentinus edodes* mycelia. Biol Pharm Bull. 2006;29(8):1651-4

144. Post-treatment of *Ganoderma lucidum* reduced liver fibrosis induced by thioacetamide in mice. Wu Y.W, Fang H.L, Lin W.C. Phytother Res. 2010;24(4):494-9

145. Pharmacological actions of gastrodia watery preparation and fermentation liquid of *Armellaria mellea* on nervous system. Chinese Journal of Medicine. 1977;(8):470-472

146. To use *Armellaria fungus* tablet to replace gastrodia tuber in treating 45 cases with syndrome of deficiency of yin and flourishing yang. Chinese Journal of Medicine. 1977;(8):473-474

147. Observation on curative effects of *Armellaria mellea* fungus tablet in treating 100 cases of neurasthenia and hypertension, etc. Zhou Linshen. Journal of New Medicine. 1978;(10):13

148. Jiangsu Provincial Cooperation Research Group on Gastrodia Tuber, Curative effects of gastrodia tuber *Armellaria* fungus tablet in treating some diseases of the nervous system, Jiangsu Journal of TCM. 1980;(1):35-37

149. The influence of *Hericium erinaceus* extract on myelination process *in vitro*. Kolotushkina E.V, Moldavan M.G, Voronin K.Y, Skibo G.G. Fiziol Zh. 2003;49(1):38-45

150. Functional recovery enhancement following injury to rodent peroneal nerve by Lion's Mane mushroom, *Hericium erinaceus* (Bull.: Fr.) Pers. (Aphyllophoromycetideae). Wong K.H, Naidu M, David R.P, Abdulla M.A, Abdullah N, Kuppusamy U.R, Sabaratnam V. Int J Med Mushr. 2009;11(2)

151. Primary study on proteomics about *Ganoderma lucidium* spores promoting survival and axon regeneration of injured spinal motor neurons in rats. Zhang W, Zeng Y.S, Wang Y, Liu W, Cheng J.J, Chen S.J. Zhong Xi Yi Jie He Xue Bao. 2006;4(3):298-302

152. Inflammatory process in Parkinson's disease: role for cytokines. Nagatsu T, Sawada M. Curr Pharm Des. 2005;11(8):999-1016

153. Dopamine- or L-DOPA-induced neurotoxicity: the role of dopamine quinone formation and tyrosinase in a model of Parkinson's disease. Asanuma M, Miyazaki I, Ogawa N. Neurotox Res. 2003;5(2):165-76

154. Parkin protects against tyrosinase-mediated dopamine neuro-toxicity by suppressing stress-activated protein kinase pathways. Hasegawa T, Treis A, Patenge N, Fiesel F.C, Springer W, Kahle P.J. J Neurochem. 2008;105(5):1700-15

155. Dopamine, in the presence of tyrosinase, covalently modifies and inactivates tyrosine hydroxylase. Xu Y : Stokes A.H : Roskoski, R: Vrana, K.E. J-Neurosci-Res. 1998;54(5):691-7

156. Tyrosinase exacerbates dopamine toxicity but is not genetically associated with Parkinson's disease. Greggio E, Bergantino E, Carter D, Ahmad R, Costin G.E, Hearing V.J, Clarimon J, Singleton A, Eerola J, Hellström O, Tienari P.J, Miller D.W, Beilina A, Bubacco L, Cookson M.R. J Neurochem. 2005;93(1):246-56

157. Oral administration of proteoglycan isolated from *Phellinus linteus* in the prevention and treatment of collagen-induced arthritis in mice. Kim G.Y, Kim S.H, Hwang S.Y, Kim H.Y, Park Y.M, Park S.K, Lee M.K, Lee S.H, Lee T.H, Lee J.D. Biol Pharm Bull. 2003;26(6):823-31

158. Study of new ways of supplementary and combinatory therapy of rheumatoid arthritis with immunomodulators. Glucomannan and Imunoglukán in adjuvant arthritis. Bauerová K, Paulovicová E, Mihalová D, Svík K, Ponist S. Toxicol Ind Health. 2009;25(4-5):329-35

159. Anti-inflammatory and anti-tumour-promoting effects of triterpene acids and sterols from the fungus *Ganoderma lucidum*. Akihisa T, Nakamura Y, Tagata M, Tokuda H, Yasukawa K, Uchiyama E, Suzuki T, Kimura Y. Chem Biodivers. 2007;4(2):224-3

160. Suppression of the inflammatory response by triterpenes isolated from the mushroom *Ganoderma lucidum*. Dudhgaonkar S, Thyagarajan A, Sliva D. Int Immunopharmacol. 2009;9(11):1272-80

161. An extract of *Antrodia camphorata* mycelia attenuates the progression of nephritis in systemic lupus Erythematosus-Prone NZB/W F1 mice. Chang J.M, Lee Y.R, Hung L.M, Liu S.Y, Kuo M.T, Wen W.C, Chen P. Evid Based Complement Alternat Med. 2008 Sep

Appendix:
Medicinal Mushrooms according to Traditional Chinese Medicine

Glossary

Index

Further Reading

APPENDIX

Medicinal Mushrooms according to Traditional Chinese Medicine

An overview of medicinal mushroom's TCM energetics is presented here in order to facilitate their use by traditionally trained practitioners.

In compiling this list I have used several sources (see list at end). Wherever possible I have used multiple sources but for *Sang Huang* and *Hou Tou Gu* I have relied exclusively on the Chinese Pharmacopoeia, 2010.

Some mushrooms are included in the main body of the text but not listed here and for these I have been unable to find reliable energetic descriptions.

Bai Mu Er/Yin Er (*Tremella fuciformis*)

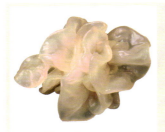

Taste - Sweet and bland

Energy - neutral

Channels Entered - Lung, Stomach (and Kidney - Hsu)

Actions - Nourishes Lung- and Stomach-Yin and treats cough due to Lung Deficiency

The actions listed above are according to contemporary materia medica. Ying et. al. add that it 'Stimulates the Heart and Nourishes the Brain, Enriches the Kidneys and Strengthens Semen', actions which find some resonance in modern research, especially its ability to benefit cardiovascular health and neurological function.

Dong Chong Xia Cao (*Cordyceps sinensis*)

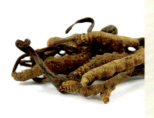

Taste - Sweet

Energy - Slightly Warm

Channels Entered - Lung and Kidney

Actions - Tonifies Kidney-Yang and Lung-Yin. Augments the Essence. Transforms Phlegm and Stops Cough

Fu Ling (*Poria cocos*)

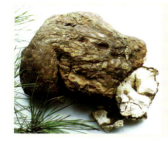

Taste - Sweet and bland

Energy - Neutral

Channels Entered - Heart, Spleen, Kidney

Actions - Promotes urination and drains Damp. Strengthens the Spleen. Calms the Shen

Fu Ling Pi, the outer skin of the sclerotium, is considered the most Damp draining and the *Fu Shen*, the innermost portion, the most calming, while *Chi Fu Ling* (the reddish portion just inside the skin) is considered to clear Heat and drain Damp.

Hou Tou Gu (*Hericium erinaceus*)

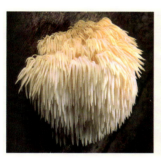

Taste - Sweet and bland

Energy - Neutral

Channels Entered - Spleen, Stomach, Heart

Actions - Strengthens the Stomach and Regulates Qi, tonifies the Spleen and promotes digestion, calms the Shen and strengthens the Brain

Ling Zhi (*Ganoderma lucidum*)

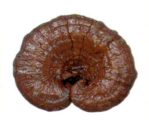

Taste - Sweet and slightly bitter

Energy - Neutral (slightly Warm - Yeung)

Channels Entered - Heart, Liver, Lung

Actions - Tonifies Qi and Nourishes Blood. Calms the Shen. Transforms Phlegm and Stops Cough

Widely considered analagous to the plant *Chi* referred to in a number of early Taoist works as a plant that brings happiness and immortality, *Ling Zhi* was originally sub-divided into 6 categories according to colour: green, red, yellow, white, black, purple.

Today's commercially available *Ling Zhi* is almost exclusively the red variety (also called Dan 'cinnabar'), which according to Hobbs is classified in the *Shen Nong Ben Cao* as having a bitter taste and acting on the Heart. This is contrary to modern materia medica, which describe *Ling Zhi* as having a sweet flavour (associated with the yellow variety in the early categorisation).

My own perception is that Ling Zhi definitely has a bitter quality (the triterpenes responsible for much of its action are extremely bitter), which correlates with its action on the Heart, and accordingly I have included bitterness in its tastes.

Mi Huan Jun (*Armillaria mellea*)

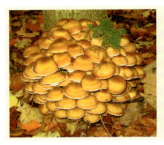

Taste - Sweet

Energy - Neutral

Channels Entered - Liver

Actions - Calms the liver to extinguish internal wind and restrain floating yang

Mu Er (*Auricularia auricula/Auricularia polytricha*)

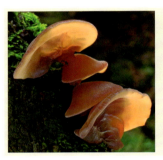

Taste - Sweet

Energy - Neutral

Channels Entered - Spleen, Liver

Actions - Enriches energy and blood, invigorates blood circulation, nourishes lungs, stops haemorrhage, invigorates bowel movement

As with *Ling Zhi*, *Mu Er* was originally sub-divided according to colour with different properties ascribed to each colour. However, today it is the black colour that is the standard type and the qualities given above are accordingly those of *Hei Mu Er* (Black Wood Ear).

Sang Huang (*Phellinus linteus*)

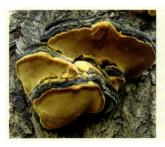

Taste - Slightly bitter

Energy - Cold

Channels Entered - Liver, Stomach, Large Intestine

Actions - Clears Damp-Heat and Stomach Fire, resolves Phlegm, invigorates Blood, stops Bleeding and relieves Pain

Xiang Gu (*Lentinus edodes*)

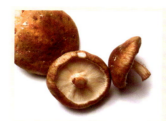

Taste - Sweet

Energy - Neutral

Channels Entered - Stomach, Spleen, Lungs

Actions - Tonifies Qi and Blood

Yun Zhi (*Trametes versicolor*)

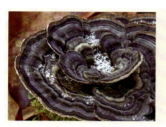

Taste - Sweet and slightly bitter

Energy - Slightly warm

Channels Entered - Lung, Liver, Spleen

Actions - Dispels Damp, reduces Phlegm, nourishes the Mind

Zhu Ling (*Polyporus umbellatus*)

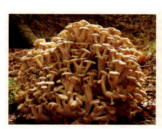

Taste - Slightly sweet

Energy - Slightly cool

Channels Entered - Spleen, Kidney, Bladder

Actions - Promotes urination and leaches out Damp

The description in Li Shi Zhen that it 'Disperses invading vicious factors and facilitates urination. Long term use makes one feel happy and vigorous and look younger' indicates that the modern usage of this mushroom is narrower than earlier.

REFERENCES

Chinese Herbal Materia Medica. Bensky D, Clavey S, Stoger E. 2004. Seattle:Eastland Press

Chinese Medical Herbology and Pharmacology. Chen JK, Chen TT. 2004. City of Industry:Art of Medicine Press

Chinese Pharmacopoeia, 2010. Beijing:Chinese Medicine Science and Technology Publishing House

Compendium of Materia Medica (Ben Cao Gang Mu). Li Shi Zhen. Tran. Luo Xiwen. 2003. Beijing:Foreign Languages Press

Handbook of Chinese Herbs. Yeung HC. 1996. Rosemead:Institute of Chinese Medicine

Icones of Medicinal Fungi from China. Ying J et al. 1987. Beijing:Science Press

Medicinal mushrooms - An Exploration of Tradition, Healing and Culture. Hobbs C. 1986. Williams:Botanica Press

Medicinal Mushrooms in TCM. Maciocia G. Mycology News. 1999;1(2):1-2

Oriental Materia Medica - A Concise Guide. Hsu HY. 1986. New Canaan:Keats Publishing Inc.

Glossary

Activator protein-1	Protein involved in the control of a number of cellular processes, including differentiation, proliferation and apoptosis.
Adjuvant	Pharmacological or immunological agent that modifies the action of other drugs or vaccines.
Akt	Akt (also called Akt1) is a protein kinase involved in cellular survival pathways by inhibiting apoptotic processes.
ALP	Alkaline phospatase - raised levels of this enzyme may be indicative of liver damage.
ALT	Alanine transferase - raised levels of this enzyme may be indicative of liver damage.
Angiogenesis	Process of blood vessel formation important in growth and development, wound-healing and tumour spread.
AP-1	See Activator protein-1.
Apoptosis	Process of programmed cell death that plays an important role in controlling cancers and viral infections.
AST	Aspartate aminotransferase - raised levels of this enzyme may be indicative of liver damage.
B-cells	Type of white blood cell that plays a major role in humoral (antibody-mediated) immunity.
Beta-glucosidase	Microbial enzyme involved in the breakdown of beta-linked polysaccharides.
Beta-glucuronidase	Enzyme involved in the breakdown of complex carbohydrates.
CCl4	Carbon tetrachloride.
Cell-signalling pathways	Chains of molecular interactions, initiated by activation of receptors on the cell surface and controlling cell processes such as gene regulation, cell proliferation and apoptosis.
Cheilitis	A medical condition involving inflammation of the lip.
Cholinergic	Related to the neutransmitter acetylcholine (the brainstem and parasympathetic nervous system are cholinergic, as are some parts of the sympathetic nervous system).
Colony-stimulating factor	Stimulates proliferation and differentiation of white blood cells.
Complement C3	Immune system protein that contributes to innate immunty.

Cytokine	Chemical messenger.
Dendritic cells	Immune cells whose main function is to process antigen material and present it to other immune cells.
DEVD	Amino acid sequence cleaved during cell death by apoptosis.
Eosinophil	Class of white blood cells involved in asthma and allergy control mechanisms.
GABA (γ-Aminobutyric acid)	Chief inhibitory neurotransmitter in the mammalian central nervous system.
Genoprotective	Helps protect DNA from damage.
Genotoxic	Capable of damaging DNA.
GGT	Gamma-glutamyltransferase - raised levels of this enzyme may be indicative of liver damage.
Glutathione peroxidase	The general name of an enzyme family whose main biological role is to protect the organism from oxidative damage.
GTP	Guanosine triphosphate - a nucleotide with an important role in signal transduction.
Gut dysbiosis	Microbial imbalance in the intestines.
HbeAg	Hepatitis B protein that is an indicator of active viral replication.
Hepatodynia	Pain in the liver.
IFN-γ	Interferon-gamma - Cytokine secreted by Th1 cells, NK cells and dendritic cells and critical for immunity against viral and bacterial infections and against cancer.
Immunomodulatory	Having an effect on the immune system.
Innate immune system	The part of the immune system that defends us against cancer and infection in a non-specific manner.
Kappa opiod receptor	Opiod receptor widely distributed in the brain, binding to which has dysphoric (mood lowering) and hallucinogenic effects.
Lectins	Sugar-binding proteins or glycoproteins with important physiological roles, including in the immune system.
Lentinan	Beta-glucan extracted from Lentinus edodes and licensed as an anti-cancer agent in Japan.
Leukopenia	Decreased number of white blood cells.
Lymphokine activated killer cell	White blood cell that has been stimulated to kill cancer cells.

Macrophages	White blood cells within tissues that phagocytose pathogens and stimulate other immune cells.
MAPK/ERK pathway	Chain of proteins that communicates a signal from a receptor on the cell surface to the DNA with effects including changes in cell division. In many cancers it is a defect in this pathway that leads to uncontrolled cell division.
Mitomycin C	Chemotherapeutic agent.
Monocyte	White blood cells that differentiate into either macrophages or dendritic cells.
Mycelium	Network of hyphae forming the vegetative part of the mushroom.
Natural killer cell	Type of white blood cells important in destroying cancer cells and virally infected cells.
Neutrophils	Phagocytic cells that are the most abundant type of white blood cell.
NF-kappaB	Protein complex that controls transcription of DNA.
NK cell	See Natural killer cell.
Nuclease	An enzyme able to cleave the bonds between nucleotide units in a DNA/RNA chain.
Nucleoside	Molecule which becomes a nucleotide on addition of a phosphate group
Nucleotide	Building block of nucleic acids (DNA/RNA).
Opsonin	A molecule that acts as a binding enhancer to facilitate phagocytosis.
P13K	Phosphatidylinositol 3-kinase - one of a family of enzymes involved in cellular functions such as growth, proliferation, differentiation, motility, survival and intracellular communication, which in turn are involved in cancer.
p53	Tumour suppressor protein important in preventing cancer.
PC12	Cell line derived from rat adrenal medulla that stops dividing and differentiates when treated with nerve growth factor.
Phagocytosis	The process by which cells engulf solid particles. Used to remove cell debris and pathogens.
Prostaglandins	Group of lipid compounds with diverse physiological actions, levels of which are elevated in inflammation.
Protein kinases	Enzymes which modify other proteins by the addition of phosphate groups and are known to regulate the majority of cellular pathways, especially those involved in signal transduction.

PSK (Polysaccharide K 'Krestin')	Japanese extract of protein-bound polysaccharides from Trametes versicolor.
PSP (Polysaccharide Peptide)	Chinese extract of protein-bound polysaccharides from Trametes versicolor.
Reticuloendothelial system	Immune cells present in secondary immune organs, such as the lymph nodes and spleen, and which are involved in mobilising the immune system against foreign antigens.
Reverse transcriptase	Enzyme involved in DNA formation.
S-adenosylhomocysteine hydrolase	Enzyme which hydrolyses S-adenosylhomocysteine to adenosine and homocysteine, high levels of which have been linked to increases in cardiovascular disease and Alzheimers Disease.
Sarcoma 180	Transplantable, non-metastasizing, connective tissue tumour used extensively in evaluation of anti-cancer activity.
Sclerotium	Underground hyphal mass forming a hard tuber-like structure in certain mushrooms.
Scopolamine	Anti-cholinergic agent that impairs memory in humans and mimics Alzheimer's Disease.
Signal transduction pathways	See Cell-signalling pathways.
Specific immune system	Also called the Adaptive Immune System. Part of the immune system that learns from challenges in order to mount a stronger response when next exposed to the same pathogen.
Sporoderm	Hard outer coating of fungal spores.
T-cells	Group of white blood cells that play a major role in cell-mediated immunity.
Teratogenic	Causing abnormalities in physiological development, especially birth defects.
Thromboembolism	Blood vessel blockage due to blood clot formation.
Triterpenes	Terpenes are oily compounds that are the major components of resins and essential oils. Triterpenes are terpenes composed of 6 isoprene units with the molecular formula $C30H48$.
Tumour necrosis factor	Also called tumor necrosis factor alpha (TNFα). Cytokine able to induce apoptosis and inhibit tumour growth and viral replication.

Index

ACE	52
Agaricus bisporus	87, 104
Agaricus blazei (see Agaricus brasiliensis)	
Agaricus brasiliensis	18, 19, **32**, 86, 87, 88, 89, 90, 99, 100, 105
Agaricus subrufescens	32
Alcohol-intoxication	36
Allergic rhinitis	**96**
Allergies	19, 21, 29, 34, 68
Alzheimers Disease	53, **96**
Angina	67
Antibiotics	30, 39, 107
Antrodia camphorata	20, 26, **36**, 84, 88, 89, 108, 110
Antrodia cinnamomea (see Antrodia camphorata)	
Anxiety	52, **107**
Arabinoxylans	28
Armillaria mellea	17, **39**, 82, 108
Aromatase	55, 86, 87
Arrythmia	**96**
Asthma	37, 45, 58, **97**
Auricularia auricula	**41**, 84, 87, 100
Auricularia polytricha	**41**
Auto-immune	24, 37, 53, 106
Avemar	28
Bacterial infection	97
Bai Hua Rong (see Inonotus obliquus)	
Bai Mu Er (see Tremella fuciformis)	
BCG	85
Ben Cao Gang Mu	14, 72
Benign prostatic hyperplasia	90, **98**
Beta-glucans	16, 17, 18, 19, 20, 21, 22, 23, 26, 28, 84
Betulinic acid	100
Bio-bran	28
Biological response modifiers	15
Biomass	26, 28
Bladder cancer	37, **85**
BPH (see Benign prostatic hyperplasia)	
Brain cancer	63, **85**
Breast cancer	37, 77, **85**
Breast-feeding	30
Button mushroom (*see Agaricus bisporus*)	
Cachexia	33, 73
Candida	29, 66, **108**
Cardiovascular health	37, 42, 44, 52
Caterpillar fungus (see Cordyceps sinensis)	
Cervical cancer	33, 77, **87**
Chaga (see Inonotus obliquus)	
Chemotherapy	82
Chi Fu Ling	116
Chitin	**20**, 99, 106
Cholesterol	65, 70, **104**
Chronic fatigue syndrome (CFS)	66, 68, **99**
Cinnamomum kanehirai	36
Cogumela del sol (see Agaricus brasiliensis)	
Colds (see Influenza)	
Colorectal cancer	77, **87**
Colostomy	27
COPD	45
Coprinus comatus	90, 101
Cordycepin	43
Cordyceps militaris	44, 106
Cordyceps sinensis	**43**, 83, 88, 89, 90, 96, 97, 100, 101, 102, 103, 106, 107, 108
Coriolus versicolor (see Trametes versicolor)	
Crohn's Disease (see Inflammatory bowel disease)	
Cs-4	44
Cytokines	24, 25
D-fraction	56, 88
Dementia	59, **100**
Dermatitis	65, 75
Diabetes	34, 45, 57, **100**
Dong Chong Xia Cao (see Cordyceps sinensis)	
Dong Gu (see Flammulina velutipes)	
Dopamine	109
EA-6	19, 49
EEM	49
Ehrlich ascites cancer	33
Endometrial cancer	33, **88**
Enokitake (*see Flammulina velutipes*)	
Enzymes	**21**
Epilepsy	40
Epstein-Barr virus	52, 99
Erectile dysfunction	**101**
Ergocalciferol	20
Ergosterol	20, 33
Erinacines	58
Eritadenine	64, 66, **104**
Ewing's Sarcoma	63
Extracts	**26**
FAHF-2	52
Fatigue	36
Flammulin	19
Flammulina velutipes	18, 19, **48**, 86, 87, 88, 90, 103, 104, 109
Fluid retention	73, **101**
Fomitopsis officinalis	87
Food allergies	49
Fu Ling (see Poria cocos)	

125

Fu Ling Pi	116
Fve	19, 49, 103
Galactose	18
GALT	23
Ganoderic acids	19
Ganoderma lucidum	14, 19, 26, **51**, 83, 84, 86, 87, 88, 89, 90, 96, 97, 98, 100, 102, 103, 104, 105, 107, 108, 109, 110
Ganoderma tsugae	97
Ganopoly	52
Gastric cancer	65, 77, **88**
Gastric ulcers	59
Gastritis	59, 88, **102**
Gastrodia elata	39
Gentamycin	45
Glioblastoma	63, 85
Glycoprotein (see proteoglycan)	
Golden oyster mushroom (see *Pleurotus citronopileatus*)	
Grifola frondosa	18, 19, 26, **56**, 83, 85, 90, 98, 101, 102, 104, 106
Grifron-D	83
Gut dysbiosis	27
Hair regrowth	73
Hakumokuji (see *Tremella fuciformis*)	
Hayfever (see Allergic rhinitis)	
Hedgehog mushroom (see *Hericium erinaceus*)	
Hen of the Woods (see *Grifola frondosa*)	56
Hepatitis B	37, 65, **102**
Hepatitis C	37, 102
Hericenones	58
Hericium erinaceus	17, 18, 20, 58, 83, 96, 98, 100, 101, 102, 108, 109
Herpes	77, **102**
Higher fungi	17
Himematsutake (see *Agaricus brasiliensis*)	
Hiratake (see *Pleurotus ostreatus*)	
HIV	49, 63, 65, 77, **103**
Hodgkins Disease	62
Hoelen (see *Poria cocos*)	
Honey mushroom (see *Armillaria mellea*)	
Hong Qu Mi (see *Monascus purpureus*)	
HPV	49, **103**
Hypertension	36, 40, 52, **105**
Hypsizygus marmoreus	49
Impotence (see Erectile dysfunction)	
Infertility	45, **105**
Inflammatory bowel disease	**106**
Influenza	**106**
Inonotus obliquus	18, 20, 26, **62**, 75, 90, 106
Insomnia	52, **107**
Jew's Ear (see *Auricularia auricula*)	
Jin Zhen Gu (see *Flammulina velutipes*)	
Kabanoanatake (see *Inonotus obliquus*)	
Kidney damage	**107**
Kikurage (see *Auricularia auricula*)	
Krestin (See PSK)	
Latent Heat	25
Lectins	19
LEM	64
Lentin	64
Lentinan	18, 23, 27, 29, 64, 72, 77, 79
Lentinula edodes (see *Lentinus edodes*)	
Lentinus edodes	18, 19, 26, **64**, 85, 87, 90, 97, 98, 104, 106, 108
Leucorrhoea	67
Leukaemia	33, 63, **88**
Ling Zhi (see *Ganoderma lucidum*)	
Ling-Zhi 8	19
Lion's Mane (see *Hericium erinaceus*)	58
Liquid fermentation	27
Liver cancer	37, 42, 44, 52, **88**
Liver disease	34, 36, 45, 52, **108**
Lovastatin	17, 68
LSIL	76
Lucidenic acids	19
Lung cancer	33, 77, **89**
Lymphoma	**89**
Maitake (see *Grifola frondosa*)	
Mannetake (see *Ganoderma lucidum*)	
MD-fraction	56, 88
ME (see CFS)	
Medulloblastoma	63, 85
Melanoma (see Skin cancer)	
Meniere's Syndrome	40, **108**
Meshimakobu (see *Phellinus linteus*)	
MGN-3	28
Monascus purpureus	66, 71, 104
Monkey-head mushroom (see *Hericium erinaceus*)	
MRSA	59, 98
Mu Er (see *Auricularia auricula*)	
Multiple Sclerosis	59, **108**
Nasopharyngeal cancer	
Nerve damage	59, 70, **109**
Neurasthenia	40
Neuroblastoma	63
Neuropathy	59
NGF (Nerve growth factor)	58
Niu Chang Chih (see *Antrodia camphorata*)	
Oesophageal cancer	57
Oestrogen	45
Oral cancer	37
Osteoporosis	45
Ovarian cancer	33, 63, **89**
Oyster mushroom (see *Pleurotus ostreatus*)	
Pancreatic cancer	**89**
Parkinson's Disease	51, **109**
Peanut allergy	51
Penicillin	17
Pharmacokinetics	24, 25

Phellinus linteus	**67**, 85, 86, 110
Phenols	**20**
Ping Gu (see *Pleurotus ostreatus*)	
Pleurotus citronopileatus	18
Pleurotus ostreatus	49, **70**, 85, 87, 90, 97, 99, 101, 104, 106
Polyphenols	20
Polyporus umbellatus	14, 26, 29, **72**, 85, 88, 101, 102
Polysaccharides	**21**
Poria cocos	14, 26, 29, **74**, 88, 90, 101
Pregnancy	30
Proflammin	49
Proteins	**19**
Prostate cancer	37, **90**
Protein-bound polysaccharides (see proteoglycan)	
Proteoglycan	18
PSK	15, 18, 27, 29, 76, 82, 85, 88, 89, 91, 102, 103
PSP	18, 76, 82, 83, 103
Radiation exposure	80
Radiotherapy	80, 82, 84
Red Yeast Rice (see *Monascus purpureus*)	
Reishi (see *Ganoderma lucidum*)	
Retained Pathogenic Factor	25
Reverse transcriptase inhibitors	44
Rheumatoid arthritis	53, 68, **110**
S.O.D. (see Superoxide dismutase)	
Sang Huang (see *Phellinus linteus*)	
Schizophyllan	23, 27
Schizophyllum commune	27, 82, 83, 87
Shiitake (see *Lentinus edodes*)	
Shirokikurage (see *Tremella fuciformis*)	
Skin cancer	**90**
SLE (Systemic Lupus erythematosus)	37, **110**
Snow Fungus (see *Tremella fuciformis*)	
Solid-state fermentation	28
Spores	27
Sterols	**20**
Stomach cancer (see Gastric cancer)	
Submerged fermentation	27
Sun Agaric (see *Agaricus brasiliensis*)	
Superoxide dismutase	21, 28, 44
Surgery	49, 84
Th1-Th2	24, 25
Tian Ma	39
Tinctures	27
Tochukas (see *Cordyceps sinensis*)	
Trametes versicolor	15, 18, 20, **76**, 85, 87, 88, 89, 99, 103, 106, 108
Transfer factors	91
Tremella fuciformis	14, 18, 19, 29, 30, **79**, 84, 101
Triterpenes	**19**, 26, 27, 51, 75, 98, 105, 107
Tyrosinase	21, 48, 51, 109
Ulcerative colitis (see Inflammatory bowel disease)	
Vaccination	19
Velutin	19
Velvet Foot (see *Flammulina velutipes*)	
Venous thromboembolism (VTE)	83
Vertigo	40
Vitamin C	56, 68, 70, 85, 91
Vitamin D2	20
Wood Ear (see *Auricularia auricula*)	
Wulingdan Pill	52
Xiang Gu (see *Lentinus edodes*)	64
Xylose	18
Yeast beta-glucan	18
Yin Er (see *Tremella fuciformis*)	
Zhu Ling (see *Polyporus umbellatus*)	

Further Reading

Medicinal mushrooms - An Exploration of Tradition, Healing and Culture.
Hobbs C. 1986. Pub. Botanica Press, Williams.

Reishi Mushroom - Herb of Spiritual Potency and Medical Wonder.
Willard T. 1990. Pub. Sylvan Press, Issaquah.

Medicinal mushrooms: their therapeutic properties and current medical usage with special emphasis on cancer treatments.
Smith J, Rowan N, Sullivan R. May 2002. Cancer Research UK. - Full report available at: *http://sci.cancerresearchuk.org/labs/med_mush/med_mush.html*

Medicinal Mushrooms: Ancient Remedies for Modern Ailments.
Halpern GM. 2002. Pub. M. Evans and Company Inc., New York.

Micoterapia: I Funghi Medicinali Nella Pratica Clinica.
Bianchi I. 2008. Pub. Nuova IPSA Editore, Palermo (Italian).

Links

www.mycotherapy.co.uk
Author's website on the therapeutic application of medicinal mushrooms

www.vitalpilze.de
Clinically oriented site and forum with English translation

www.healing-mushrooms.net
Website dedicated to investigating bioactive compounds from fungi

www.begellhouse.com/journals/708ae68d64b17c52.html
International Journal of Medicinal Mushrooms

www.mushroomcompany.com
For those interested in cultivating medicinal mushrooms or locating growers.

www.fungiphoto.com
Extensive library of mushroom photos